DIRECTED
ACTIVITIES

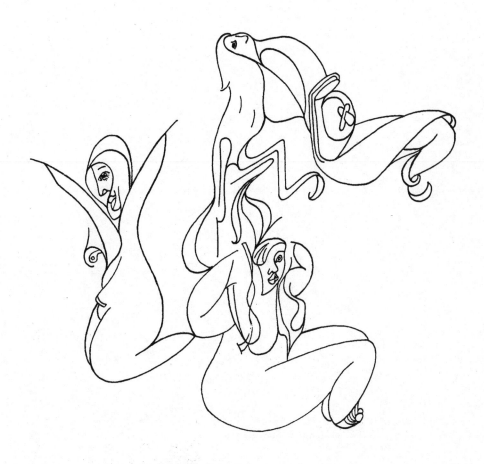

GERARD GRENNELL

DIRECTED
ACTIVITIES

A DIARY OF PRACTICAL PROCEDURES
FOR STUDENTS AND TEACHERS OF THE
F.M. ALEXANDER TECHNIQUE
AS TAUGHT AT
THE CONSTRUCTIVE TEACHING CENTRE (1989-1992)

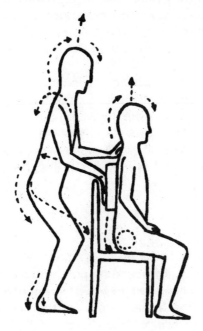

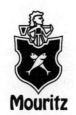

Mouritz

First published May 2002

Mouritz
6 Ravenslea Road
London SW12 8SB
Great Britain

www.mouritz.co.uk

ISBN 0–9525574–5–2   Hardback

British Library Cataloguing-in-Publication Data
A catalogue record for this book is
available from the British Library.

Printed on 80 gsm Antique White Wove
and bound in Balacron with The Bath Press, Avon.

ACKNOWLEDGEMENTS
I would like to express my most sincere gratitude to Bernie Tonge for her unfailing encouragment, advice and support, without which I could never have maintained the momentum or belief necessary for such a project. I would also like to thank Miriam Wohl for the invaluable insight and knowledge she so selflessly provided.

Gerry Grennell
March 2002

ABOUT THE AUTHOR
Since graduating from the Constructive Teaching Centre in 1992, Gerard Grennell has worked as an Alexander Technique teacher, voice coach and musician, predominantly in the film industry, both at home and abroad. He lives in Dublin, Ireland.

CONTENTS ~

PART THREE (THIRD YEAR).

TERM ONE (FIRST HALF).

TERM ONE (SECOND HALF).

FOREWORD ~

These notes of directed activities were made by Gerard Grennell between 1989 and 1992, while he was a student on Walter and Dilys Carrington's teacher training course.

A directed activity is the application of the Alexander Technique to a simple, usually small movement which will encourage length and expansion of the whole body. The movements have been selected for their ability to encourage length and width. Many of the activities are "hands-on" procedures, while others may be performed by a pupil under the supervision of a teacher, for example lifting an arm. These notes include the directed activities (often called "procedures") that Alexander developed: sitting down, standing up, "monkey", whispered ah, coming up on the toes, and hands on the back of the chair. Like Alexander's procedures, the directed activities developed by the Carringtons may appear misleadingly simple, but the simplest of activities can be very demanding when attending to the means-whereby. Much consideration and experience have gone into the development of these activities. At the time Grennell made his notes, Walter and Dilys Carrington had been teaching directed activities for thirty years. They still spend half an hour each day working on a directed activity, demonstrating the activity with a student, after which each student is taken through the activity by a teacher.

Grennell's notes and clear drawings succinctly record each directed activity. I can vouch for the accuracy of his notes, as I was there for some of the time he trained. It is crucial to remember, however, that they were created as *aides-mémoire* for those who went through the directed activities as they were presented then. This is his diary, which means it is a record of subjective impressions made at the time. Furthermore, there are shortcomings inherent in writing about how to put the Technique into practice. These shortcomings apply to all books on the Technique which contain what can easily be misconstrued as "what to do" exercises, and they need to be discussed.

What is not mentioned here is, firstly, that every activity should be preceded by the primary directions of releasing the neck, allowing the head to go forward and up, lengthening and widening the back, and sending the knees forward and away. This is a rehearsal in paying attention to the primary directions which take care of the primary control while performing an activity. What is practised is not the mere physical performance of a movement (achieving a particular goal or "end"), but the inhibition of performing a movement in a habitual manner while maintaining the directions for the new use. The student is not being asked to "do" something for the purpose of gaining a specific "end", but for the purposes of inhibiting and directing.

Secondly, very few of the activities are at first performed in their entirety. Most activities are broken down into a series of progressive steps: each day a new step is added, and so there is a gradual build-up towards the complete activity. Taking time is of the essence.

Thirdly, it is important to remember that these directed activities are initially carried out with the assistance of a teacher. The teacher checks that the primary control is working optimally at the moment preceding any attempt to move. When the student starts to move and continues to move, the teacher is able to see whether the workings of the primary control are interfered with and informs the student accordingly. The student is then less likely to get distracted or misdirect, and is in a much better position to attempt the activity without the assistance of a teacher.

In addition, the teacher who is providing the stimulus (e.g. "I want you to ...") can simultaneously monitor the student's reaction and check that the student can meet the stimulus with inhibition and direction. If the stimulus is too strong and the head-neck-back relationship is interfered with, the teacher can moderate the stimulus so that it is less likely to provoke a wrong reaction. It is part of the teacher's art to find an appropriate stimulus for each individual pupil, in a setting which is supportive and non-threatening. The teacher demands just enough to tax the student's attention and power of inhibition and direction, yet is not so demanding that the student is unlikely to accomplish the activity. Pragmatic, not dogmatic, is the attitude of the teacher who is taking a student through these activities.

This individualistic approach is a fundamental characteristic of the Technique. The analysis and feedback provided by a teacher cannot be reproduced in a book. Alexander referred to this in *Man's Supreme Inheritance*: "It would be impossible, however, to describe the method in full detail in this place, owing to the extraordinary variability of the cases presented, no two of which exhibit precisely the same defects."[1]

The fact that there cannot be a uniform set of instructions for everybody means that the whole undertaking is a matter of experimentation. As the teacher cannot know in advance how the pupil will respond to the instructions, teaching will always include elements of investigation and discovery. Both teacher and student are engaged in a process which is akin to the scientific method of predicting and testing and of learning from what goes wrong. John Dewey perceptively described it as a "process of simultaneous development of principles and consequences, used as means for testing each other."[2]

This is the fourth (and perhaps most fundamental) point concerning these activities: they are about learning how to learn, about nurturing a mental attitude of exploration and discovery. This book does not constitute an attempt to create a finite set of directed activities to be carried out stereotypically. The activities here are works in progress, and this book therefore contains a snapshot of work which, as Dewey wrote, "will no more arrive at a stage of finished perfection than does any genuine experimental scientific procedure."[3] This is also in the nature of individual growth and development: we teach according to our experiences, and as improvement in use increases, our teaching changes. The teaching of the Technique is a skill which cannot be captured as an itinerary. Growth and development have to be part of a creative process of exploration and discovery: to anticipate the result in advance is to prejudice the process.

If we are not creative, curious, or at least open to the new, we risk interpreting and practising the Technique in terms of what we already know and have experienced, and it then becomes difficult to set up a situation in which we can have a new experience and thereby gain a new understanding. When approaching an activity we have habitual ideas about what we can and cannot do, and how to go about doing it. The purpose of applying the Technique to an activity in an experimental setting is to test those ideas, to question them and, perhaps, to prove them wrong. Being right merely confirms what we already know or expect; being wrong provides us with more information: about the means-whereby one is using to gain an end, and about one's actions and reactions to a given stimulus. An experimental outlook can circumvent habit, in that it permits three things we habitually avoid: making mistakes, feeling wrong, and having new and unfamiliar experiences.

To permit oneself to make mistakes is to give oneself the stimulus of "failing" and of not reacting in a habitual way. If mistakes are expected and studied, they need not destroy courage. Instead, the experience becomes a means-whereby from which we can learn. For Alexander it was a positive experience:

> Personally, I always enjoy finding out when I have been wrong as the admission is so often a valuable experience, for it is the means-whereby to a lasting impression that tends to prevent repetition of the faulty thinking that led one into error.[4]

To permit oneself to feel wrong (which is often different from *being* wrong) is fundamental to the Technique. When feeling right is associated with habitual activity, feeling wrong becomes essential for change. Here the inhibition of "trying to be right" is paramount: getting it right by "doing" of any kind is like having the right answer to the wrong question.

To permit oneself to have a truly new experience is dependent on not making snap judgements, classifying an experience as either right or wrong (or good or bad). It is dependent on allowing for the possibility that something completely new and unknown may feel neither wrong nor right, just unfamiliar.

This is partly why experimentation does not come easily to most of us: there is no instant certainty in the process. Inhibition is needed for all of the above; inhibition extends well beyond dealing with the stimulus of performing a movement.

The beauty of the directed activities developed by Walter and Dilys is that they are so simple that mistakes are rarely a result of the movement required but rather are due to a lack of inhibition and direction (i. e. misdirection) which precede the activity. Success becomes a measure of preparation. ("Prior preparation prevents poor performance.") The preparation, the setting up of the directed activity, is the real test. Conscious preparation (as opposed to trial and error) means working out rationally and intelligently the best way to go about achieving the desired "end".

Having established the primary and secondary directions required, one continues rehearsing them throughout the performance of the activity, and only *afterwards* evaluates the performance. Generally, one's judgement of whether or not things are going badly should not be allowed to interfere with the experiment, as any instant "correction" (often carried out according to feeling) would invalidate the experiment. Any corrections or ideas for improvement should be incorporated into a new experiment: the same activity, but with added thought and inhibition where needed.

In practice the process may not be as bare or as unambiguous as this; the method may be scientific, but it is carried out by people for people with all the failings and idiosyncrasies typical of the individual. Conscious control cannot guarantee perfection: experience, emotion, motivation, etc. enter into the process, which in practice makes it more an art than a science. Because we are human, directed activities should not be approached with an attitude of clinical detachment. Walter Carrington calls directed activities "games" because he realised very early "that people ought to approach this part of the proceedings in a non-endgaining way."[5] They are called "games" because a playful attitude is much more helpful than a serious attitude.

With the above provisos in mind, I can heartily recommend this book for teachers of the Technique. Grennell's text and drawings provide an excellent primer, and much of the material here is an ideal springboard for further exploration and discovery. These games have taken Alexander's existing procedures for learning to apply the Technique to every kind of activity and expanded upon them. It is now the reader's turn to develop, as John Dewey's wrote of Alexander's technique, the "experimental procedure" and produce "new material for observation and thorough analysis."[6]

Jean M. O. Fischer
London, January 2002

1 F. M. Alexander *Man's Supreme Inheritance* (Mouritz, 1996, London) p. 132.
2 F. M. Alexander *Constructive Conscious Control of the Individual* (STAT Books, 1997, London) p. 18.
3 *Ibid*, p. 18.
4 F. M. Alexander letter to Mungo and Sydney Douglas, undated, about 1950.
5 Walter Carrington *Personally Speaking* (Mouritz, 2001, London) p. 21.
6 F. M. Alexander *Constructive Conscious Control of the Individual*, p. 18.
7 F. M. Alexander *The Use of the Self* (Chaterson, 1946, London) p. 55.
8 F. M. Alexander *The Universal Constant in Living* (Mouritz, 2000, London) p. 79.

PART ONE

TERMS ONE TWO AND THREE COMBINED

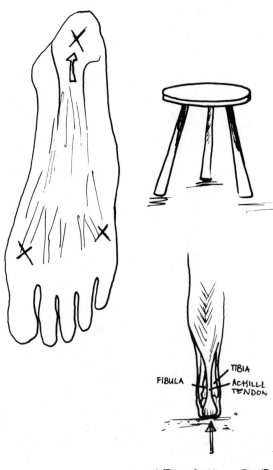

WEIGHT-BEARING POINT

FIBULA
TIBIA
ACHILLE TENDON

· STABILITY LIKE THAT OF THREE-LEGGED STOOLS

THINK OF EACH FOOT AS BEING LIKE A THREE-LEGGED STOOL — WITH ONE POINT AT THE HEEL — ANOTHER AT THE BASE OF YOUR LITTLE TOE — AND ANOTHER AT THE BASE OF YOUR BIG TOE — YET THE HEELS BEARING MOST OF THE WEIGHT...

ALLOW YOUR TOES TO FEEL THE FLOOR AS THOUGH THEY WERE FINGERS...

STANDING WITH YOUR FEET UNDER YOUR HIPS — THINK OF THE FLOOR COMING UP TO THE FEET, AND THE SENSE OF WEIGHT ON THE HEELS PROVIDING THE STIMULUS TO LENGTHEN IN STATURE, OR TO GO UP.

BE CAREFUL NOT TO STAND WITH YOUR FEET TOO FAR APART — OTHERWISE YOUR WEIGHT WILL TEND TO "DROP" THROUGH THE MIDDLE AS YOU TENSE THE OUTSIDE OF THE LEGS, AND, IF TOO CLOSE TOGETHER, YOU WILL BE CONSTANTLY WORKING TO HOLD YOUR BODY UPRIGHT (USING EXCESSIVE EFFORT).

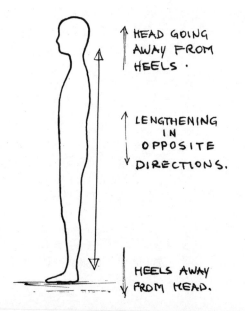

HEAD GOING AWAY FROM HEELS.

LENGTHENING IN OPPOSITE DIRECTIONS.

HEELS AWAY FROM HEAD.

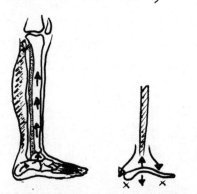

WEIGHT PROVIDES STIMULUS FOR "UP"!

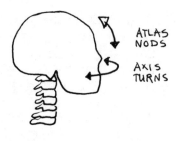

ATLAS
NODS

AXIS
TURNS

MORE WEIGHT
TO THE FRONT

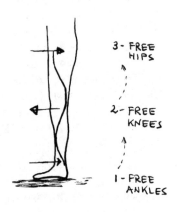

3 - FREE
HIPS

2 - FREE
KNEES

1 - FREE
ANKLES

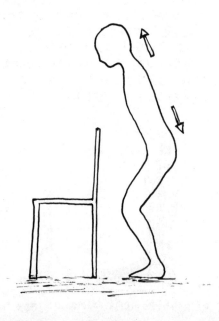

• MONKEY (POSITION OF MECHANICAL ADVANTAGE)

YOUR HEAD HAS MORE WEIGHT TO THE FRONT THAN TO THE BACK (IT IS BALANCED JUST BEHIND THE EARS), THEREFORE THE TENDENCY TO NOD FORWARD IS ALREADY THERE — BUT, TO COMPENSATE, WE PULL OUR HEADS BACK, BY SHORTENING OUR NECK MUSCLES, AND IN·TURN, PLACING STRAIN ON THE SPINE, EVENTUALLY DISTORTING IT.

NOD FORWARD AND YOU WILL FALL FORWARD - UNLESS YOU COMPENSATE BY COMING BACK ON TO YOUR HEELS. NOD BACK - OR PULL YOUR HEAD BACK - AND YOU WILL HAVE TO COME ON TO YOUR TOES.

GOING INTO MONKEY, THINK OF THE FLOOR COMING UP TO YOUR FEET.

EYES NOT FIXED (STARING TENDS TO FIX US) SO FIND SOMETHING TO LOOK AT,

DIRECTING—

ANKLES FREE...
KNEES FREE...
HIPS FREE...
DROP YOUR NOSE SLIGHTLY (NOD, OR ROLL, YOUR HEAD) AND GO INTO MONKEY---

REMAIN ONLY FOR AS LONG AS IS COMFORTABLE - BUILDING ON GOOD EXPERIENCE.

· HANDS ON THE BACK OF A
CHAIR (AND ULNAR DEVIATION)

GO INTO MONKEY AS DESCRIBED
AND ONCE IN MONKEY
REMEMBER THAT YOU HAVE
PROBABLY TIGHTENED AS A
RESULT OF MOVING, SO ASK
FOR LENGTH AGAIN

KEEPING YOUR FINGERS TOGETHER
OPEN BOTH HANDS OUT BY
STRAIGHTENING THE FINGERS
AS THOUGH YOU WERE POINTING
TO THE FLOOR

SLOWLY BRING EACH HAND UP
(ONE AT A TIME) TO REST ON
THE BACK OF THE CHAIR IN
FRONT OF YOU (PALMS FACING
UPWARDS)

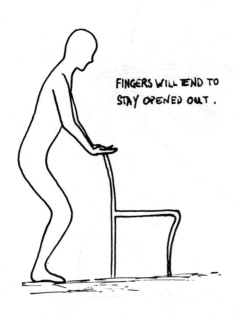

FINGERS WILL TEND TO
STAY OPENED OUT.

YOU MAY NOTICE THAT IN THIS POSITION YOUR WRISTS ARE
BENT AND THE FINGERS POINTING SLIGHTLY TOWARDS
EACH OTHER — THIS IS CALLED "ULNAR DEVIATION" AND WILL
NECESSITATE A DEEPER MONKEY TO REDUCE IT, BECAUSE
OUR ELBOWS POINT OUTWARDS (AWAY FROM THE BODY) AND
CLOSE THE SHOULDERS

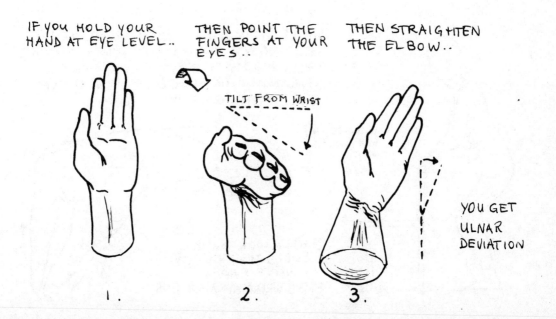

IF YOU HOLD YOUR
HAND AT EYE LEVEL..

THEN POINT THE
FINGERS AT YOUR
EYES..

THEN STRAIGHTEN
THE ELBOW..

TILT FROM WRIST

YOU GET
ULNAR
DEVIATION

1.   2.   3.

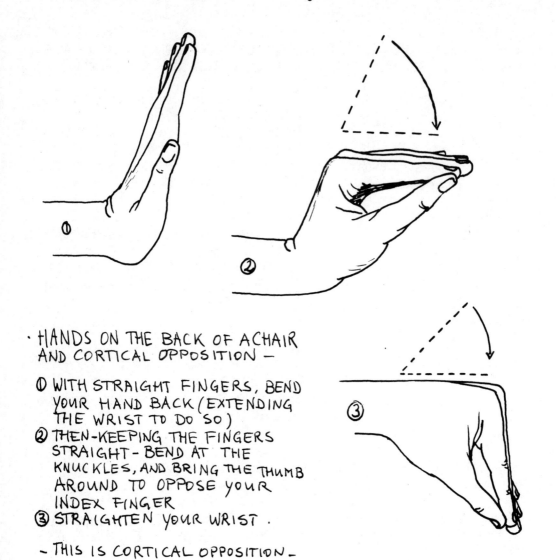

· HANDS ON THE BACK OF A CHAIR
AND CORTICAL OPPOSITION —

① WITH STRAIGHT FINGERS, BEND
   YOUR HAND BACK (EXTENDING
   THE WRIST TO DO SO)
② THEN—KEEPING THE FINGERS
   STRAIGHT—BEND AT THE
   KNUCKLES, AND BRING THE THUMB
   AROUND TO OPPOSE YOUR
   INDEX FINGER
③ STRAIGHTEN YOUR WRIST .

— THIS IS CORTICAL OPPOSITION —

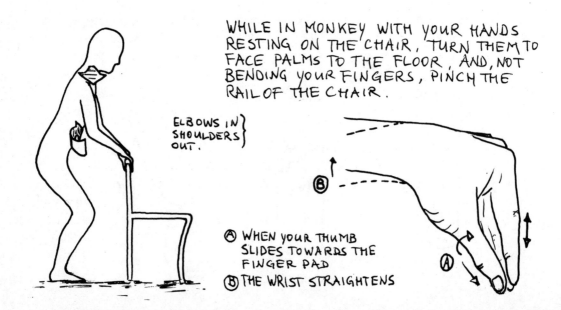

WHILE IN MONKEY WITH YOUR HANDS
RESTING ON THE CHAIR, TURN THEM TO
FACE PALMS TO THE FLOOR , AND, NOT
BENDING YOUR FINGERS, PINCH THE
RAIL OF THE CHAIR.

ELBOWS IN }
SHOULDERS }
OUT.

Ⓐ WHEN YOUR THUMB
   SLIDES TOWARDS THE
   FINGER PAD
Ⓑ THE WRIST STRAIGHTENS

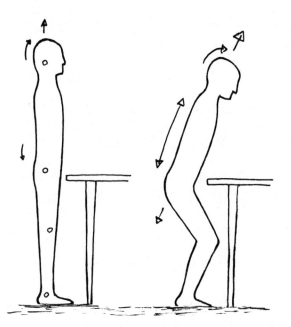

MONKEY – WITH HANDS ON THE TEACHING TABLE.

STANDING WITH A GOOD SUPPORTING DISTANCE BETWEEN YOUR TWO FEET.

LENGTHENING AND WIDENING – GO INTO MONKEY... AND NOW THAT YOU HAVE MOVED – CHECK YOUR DIRECTIONS AGAIN, BECAUSE IT IS LIKELY THAT YOU HAVE TIGHTENED IN SOME WAY.

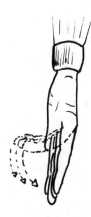

WITH YOUR ARMS DOWN BY YOUR SIDE – OPEN YOUR HANDS BY POINTING YOUR FINGERS TO THE FLOOR.

THEN – BY BENDING YOUR ELBOWS BACK – BRING EACH HAND (SEPARATELY) UP TO REST ON THE TABLE PALMS DOWN... ONCE AGAIN – CHECK YOUR DIRECTIONS.

NOW COME (FORWARD AND UP) OVER ON TO YOUR HANDS – TAKING ABOUT HALF YOUR WEIGHT ON YOUR ARMS AND INTO YOUR BACK ... SOFTEN YOUR NECK AND GIVE YOUR DIRECTIONS.

YOU CAN NOW LOOK TO RELEASE YOUR BOTTOM AWAY FROM YOUR HEAD, AND FREE YOUR KNEES FORWARD WITH LENGTH IN THE THIGHS – FREE ANKLES AND LENGTHEN UP THE FRONT.

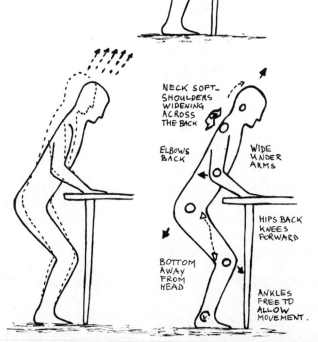

NECK SOFT – SHOULDERS WIDENING ACROSS THE BACK

ELBOWS BACK

WIDE UNDER ARMS

HIPS BACK KNEES FORWARD

BOTTOM AWAY FROM HEAD

ANKLES FREE TO ALLOW MOVEMENT.

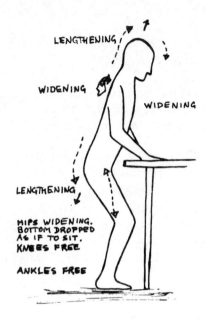

LENGTHENING

WIDENING

WIDENING

LENGTHENING

HIPS WIDENING.
BOTTOM DROPPED
AS IF TO SIT.
KNEES FREE

ANKLES FREE

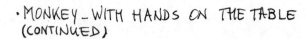

· MONKEY – WITH HANDS ON THE TABLE
(CONTINUED)

WHEN YOU SENSE A MOVEMENT, OR
JUST A FEELING THAT THERE IS
A RESPONSE TO YOUR REQUEST
FOR YOUR THIGHS TO LENGTHEN
WHILE YOUR HANDS ARE ON THE
TABLE, YOU CAN THEN APPLY THE
SAME PROCEDURE OF REQUESTING
LENGTH IN YOUR THIGHS WHILE
IN MONKEY (WITH YOUR HANDS NOT
TAKING WEIGHT)

THEN COME INTO UPRIGHT.

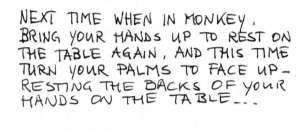

NEXT TIME WHEN IN MONKEY,
BRING YOUR HANDS UP TO REST ON
THE TABLE AGAIN, AND THIS TIME
TURN YOUR PALMS TO FACE UP –
RESTING THE BACKS OF YOUR
HANDS ON THE TABLE...

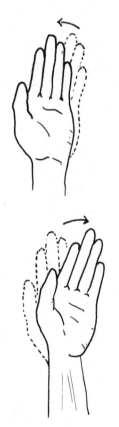

YOUR HANDS WILL TEND TO PULL
INWARDS ON THE ULNAR SIDE (
LITTLE FINGER SIDE), SO BRING
THEM BACK OUT (AS BEST YOU
CAN) WITHOUT TIGHTENING,
YOU MAY NOTICE YOUR ELBOWS
HUGGING THE SIDES OF YOUR
CHEST – ASK FOR WIDTH ACROSS
THE UPPER ARMS (AND ARMPITS).

NOW BRING YOUR WEIGHT GENTLY
OVER ON TO YOUR HANDS.
AGAIN, YOUR HANDS MAY PULL
TO THE ULNAR SIDE (BECAUSE, AS
YOU COME OVER ON TO YOUR
HANDS, YOUR WRISTS WILL BEND
A LITTLE MORE AND BRING
ABOUT ULNAR DEVIATION)

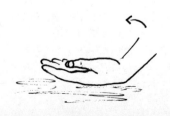

· HANDS ON THE TABLE (CONTINUED).

IN THIS POSITION, THE MORE ACUTE THE ANGLE OF THE WRISTS, THE MORE ACUTE THE ULNAR DEVIATION WILL BE, WITH THE RESULT THAT THE ELBOWS MAY POINT OUT AND AWAY FROM THE SIDES, AND THE SHOULDERS NARROW

(HANDS POINTING IN — ELBOWS OUT — SHOULDERS IN)...

THE CLOSER YOUR HANDS ARE (TO EACH OTHER) THE GREATER THE ANGLE WILL APPEAR, AND THE MORE YOUR ELBOWS MAY TEND TO POINT OUTWARDS FROM YOUR SIDES.

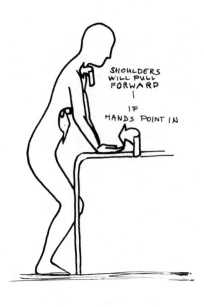

SHOULDERS WILL PULL FORWARD
IF HANDS POINT IN

LENGTH IN THE LOWER ARM. IT IS DESIRABLE TO BE ABLE TO STRAIGHTEN (OR REDUCE THE ANGLE OF TURN-IN) AND APART FROM THE ALREADY-MENTIONED DEEPER MONKEY, YOU WILL HAVE TO LOOK FOR YOUR SHOULDERS TO WIDEN, WHICH WILL THEN BRING THE ELBOWS MORE IN TO THE SIDES. ONLY THEN WILL YOU BE ABLE TO BEGIN ASKING FOR LENGTH BETWEEN YOUR WRIST AND ELBOW, OR SENDING YOUR ELBOW AWAY FROM YOUR HAND (AND WRIST).

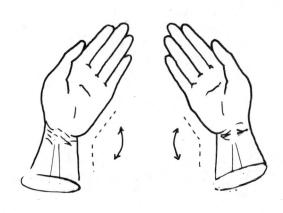

ROTATE YOUR THUMB ON AN AXIS AROUND THE LITTLE FINGER — ROLLING FROM THE WRIST

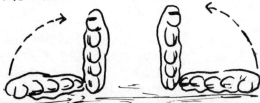

TO BRING YOUR HANDS ONTO THEIR SIDES —
ONCE SATISFIED WITH THE ABOVE, TURN YOUR HANDS (ONE AT A TIME AT FIRST) ON TO THEIR SIDES (PALMS FACING EACH OTHER)

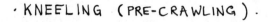

· KNEELING (PRE-CRAWLING) ·

STANDING AT FIRST — BEGIN BY
ALLOWING THE WEIGHT ON YOUR
HEELS TO GIVE YOU THE STIMULUS
TO GO UP (LENGTHEN IN STATURE)...

THEN COME BACK A LITTLE BIT
MORE ON TO YOUR HEELS, AND
PLACE ONE FOOT BEHIND THE
OTHER (BENDING THAT KNEE)....

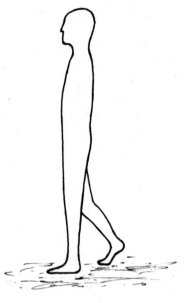

TAKING YOUR TIME, LOWER YOURSELF
ON TO THE KNEE BEHIND YOU.
(YOU MAY FIND YOUR FORWARD
FOOT RAISED, BUT THAT IS O.K.).
DO NOT RUSH AHEAD: INSTEAD — GET
YOUR BALANCE FROM THE KNEE
ON THE FLOOR AND YOUR FORWARD
FOOT...(HEEL)...

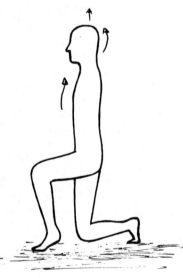

NOW YOU CAN BRING YOUR OTHER
KNEE TO THE FLOOR, MAKING
SURE THAT THERE IS ENOUGH
DISTANCE BETWEEN EACH KNEE
TO SUPPORT EACH HIP —
I.E. KNEES UNDER PELVIS.

YOUR FEET SHOULD NOT BE
FALLING OUT FROM SIDE TO
SIDE — AND AT THIS POINT YOU
MAY ALSO WANT TO EXTEND
THEM.

· RELEASE UPWARDS
LOOKING FOR FREE-
DOM IN YOUR LEGS,
HIPS, BOTTOM, SPINE,
(NECK) AND ANKLES

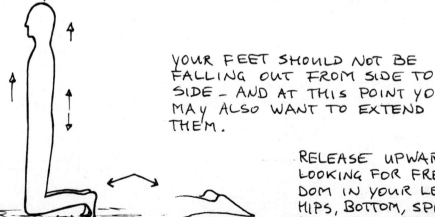

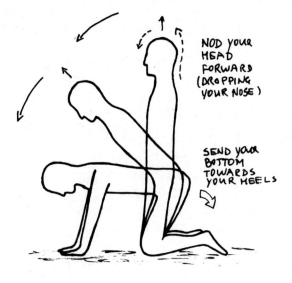

NOD YOUR HEAD FORWARD (DROPPING YOUR NOSE)

SEND your BOTTOM TOWARDS YOUR HEELS

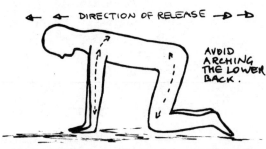

← ← DIRECTION OF RELEASE → ▷ ▷

AVOID ARCHING THE LOWER BACK.

WEIGHT EVEN - HANDS UNDER SHOULDERS
KNEES UNDER HIPS (AND SOFT NECK)

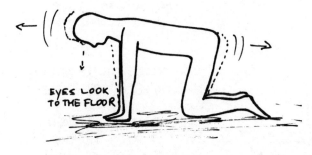

← ROCKING GENTLY →

EYES LOOK TO THE FLOOR

• CRAWLING (ROCKING)

ONCE ON BOTH KNEES YOU WILL NOW WANT TO COME ON TO BOTH HANDS. THIS CAN BE ACHIEVED BY NODDING YOUR HEAD FORWARD, AND ALSO SENDING YOUR BOTTOM BACK (BENDING AT THE HIP JOINTS). GENTLY RESTING ON YOUR HANDS. DIRECT YOUR HEAD FORWARD TO BRING YOUR BODY WITH IT.
CAREFUL NOT TO COME DOWN-- ON TO YOUR HANDS: INSTEAD- COME GRADUALLY OVER AND ON TO THEM. THUS KEEPING THE WEIGHT FROM SUDDENLY COMING ON TO YOUR SHOULDERS CAUSING THEM TO NARROW AND TIGHTEN. THEN WITH YOUR SHOULDERS ABOVE YOUR WRISTS, AND YOUR HIPS ABOVE YOUR KNEES, DISTRIBUTE YOUR WEIGHT EVENLY, CAREFUL NOT TO DROP YOUR WAIST TOWARDS THE FLOOR.
SOFTEN YOUR NECK- ALLOWING YOUR HEAD TO GO AWAY FROM YOUR BOTTOM AND YOUR BOTTOM AWAY FROM YOUR HEAD — SOFTEN BEHIND YOUR KNEES, AND YOUR HEAD STARTS YOU ROCKING GENTLY FORWARD AND BACK.

YOUR HEAD PULLS THE REST OF YOUR BODY WITH IT WHILE THE HIPS DO THE SAME THING - CONSTANTLY MAINTAINING THE DISTANCE OR LENGTH BETWEEN THEM.

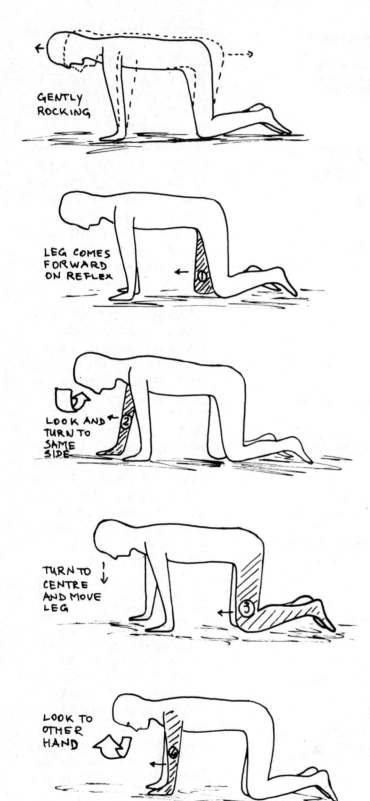

GENTLY
ROCKING

LEG COMES
FORWARD
ON REFLEX

①

LOOK AND
TURN TO
SAME
SIDE

②

TURN TO
CENTRE
AND MOVE
LEG

③

LOOK TO
OTHER
HAND

④

· CRAWLING (CONTINUED).

FOUR-FOUR TIME ($\frac{4}{4}$) OR SAME-SIDE LEG AND ARM — ONE AFTER THE OTHER, FOLLOWED BY THE OTHER LEG AND THEN SAME-SIDE ARM, USING YOUR EYES TO TURN YOUR HEAD TO THE SIDE YOU MOVE — (BY LOOKING AT THAT HAND)...

BEGIN BY GENTLY ROCKING TO AND FRO, THEN CHOOSE ONE OF THE FORWARD ROCKS TO GO A LITTLE BIT FURTHER FORWARD, ALLOWING IT TO ACTIVATE THE REFLEX THAT MOVES YOUR THIGH FORWARD, THUS ACCOMMODATING THE SENSE OF FALLING FORWARD — (DO NOT LIFT THE KNEE — SLIDE IT)...

LOOK AT THE SAME-SIDE HAND (ALSO TURN HEAD) WHILE BRINGING IT FORWARD AT THE SAME TIME...

WHILE LOOKING TO THE FLOOR, BRING YOUR OTHER LEG ALONGSIDE THE FIRST...

CONTINUE ON THROUGH TO LOOK AT THE NEXT HAND WHILE AT THE SAME TIME BRINGING THAT HAND FORWARD TO ALONGSIDE THE OTHER — GRADUALLY INCREASING SPEED.

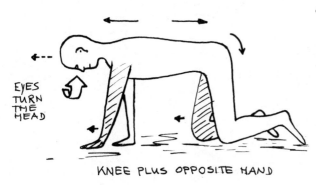

EYES TURN THE HEAD

KNEE PLUS OPPOSITE HAND

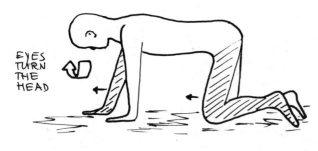

EYES TURN THE HEAD

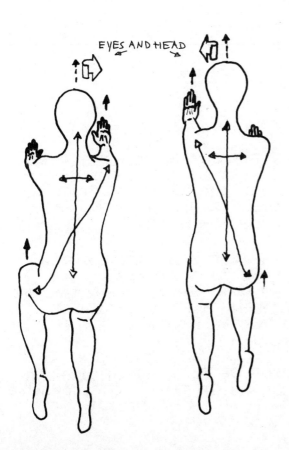

EYES AND HEAD

• CRAWLING (CONTINUED).

THIS TIME TRY CROSS PATTERN, IN OTHER WORDS, A KNEE AND THE OPPOSITE HAND.

BEGIN BY FOLLOWING THE PROCEDURE AT THE BEGINNING OF PREVIOUS PAGE, THEN FOLLOW THROUGH (AS A REFLEX) WITH ONE LEG. AND AS SOON AS THAT LEG MOVES, LIFT THE OPPOSITE HAND, AND BRING THE WEIGHT ON TO BOTH AT THE SAME TIME. THE KNEE LEADS— KNEE SLIDES AND THEN THE HAND LIFTS—BUT BOTH COME DOWN AT THE SAME TIME. THIS IS TO STOP THE HAND GOING FIRST AND MAKING TOO BIG A GAP BETWEEN KNEE AND HAND, THEN CARRY ON USING THE OTHER ARM AND LEG. ALSO TRY USING SAME-SIDE LIMBS TOGETHER.

LOOKING AT THE FORWARD HAND IS NOT DONE BY SWIMMERS FOR EXAMPLE. THEY TURN AND BREATHE ON THE BACK-HAND SIDE.

HORSES DO NOT TURN TO THE FORWARD SIDE EITHER.

AS YOU MOVE — NECK SOFTENING AND FREE, HEAD FORWARD AND OUT, BOTTOM DIRECTED AWAY FROM HEAD, SPINE LENGTHENING, SHOULDERS AND HIPS WIDENING.

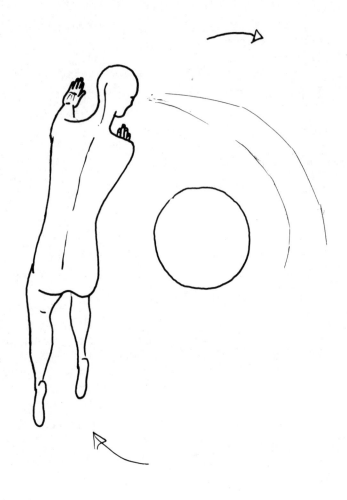

· CRAWLING IN A CIRCLE (AROUND AN OBJECT).

FIRST — SET YOURSELF UP FOR CRAWLING AS BEFORE,
THEN — LOOKING IN THE DIRECTION YOU INTEND TO GO
(AS IF LOOKING AROUND THE CORNER AT AN IMAGINARY
PATHWAY), YOUR EYES WILL LEAD YOUR HEAD, AND
YOUR HEAD WILL LEAD YOUR SPINE.

THE INSIDE LEG AND ARM HAVE A SHORTER STRIDE
RELATIVE TO THE OUTSIDE LEG AND ARM. YOU
WILL ALSO NOTICE THAT YOUR SPINE SHORTENS ON
THE INSIDE AND LENGTHENS ON THE OUTSIDE
(THINK OF THE CURVE AS BEING FROM YOUR
BOTTOM TO YOUR HEAD)

WHEN CRAWLING TO A COUNT OF FOUR, BEGIN WITH THE
INSIDE KNEE, FIRST CLOCKWISE THEN ANTICLOCKWISE.
YOU WILL PROBABLLY HAVE A DOMINANT SIDE, SO
OBSERVE WHICH SIDE YOU FAVOUR.

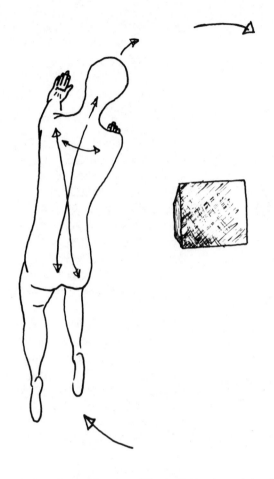

• CRAWLING (CONTINUED).

THIS TIME TRY CRAWLING AROUND AN OBJECT WITHOUT TURNING THE HEAD (ON THE AXIS) IN THE DIRECTION YOU ARE GOING. INSTEAD- NOD YOUR HEAD TO THE SIDE (OF THE DIRECTION IN WHICH YOU ARE GOING). THIS WILL BEND THE NECK SIMILAR TO THE WAY A HORSE WOULD, WHILE WALKING IN A CIRCLE.
OBSERVE THE RESULT.

OTHER PATTERNS OF CRAWLING ARE ...
① SAME SIDE, FOUR TIME. (KNEE-HAND-KNEE-HAND)
② SAME SIDE TWO TIME. (KNEE AND HAND TOGETHER)
③ OPPOSITES, FOUR TIME. (RIGHT KNEE-LEFT HAND)
④ OPPOSITES, TWO TIME. (OPPOSITES TOGETHER).

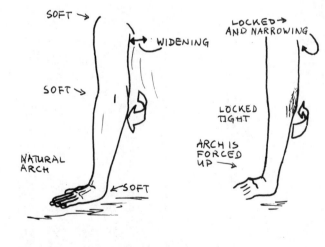

SOFT →
WIDENING
SOFT →
NATURAL ARCH
← SOFT

LOCKED → AND NARROWING
LOCKED TIGHT
ARCH IS FORCED UP →

IF YOUR ARMS ARE TIGHTENING TO TAKE THE WEIGHT - THE ELBOWS WILL TEND TO POINT OR PULL INTO THE SIDES - BUT NOT SO IF THEY ARE SPRINGY...

KEEP YOUR FINGERS TOGETHER, AND THIS WILL HELP KEEP THE HAND ARCHED... AVOID GRIPPING IN THE FINGERS... YOUR FINGERS WILL EVENTUALLY START TO STRAIGHTEN OUT (DONT RUSH IT).

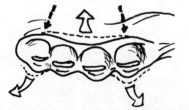

GENTLE PRESSURE ON THE OUTSIDES OF THE HANDS WILL LIFT AND WIDEN THEM

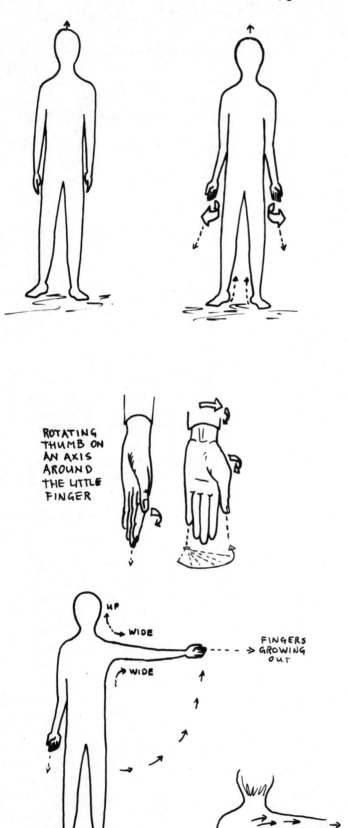

ROTATING
THUMB ON
AN AXIS
AROUND
THE LITTLE
FINGER

UP
WIDE
FINGERS
→ GROWING
OUT
WIDE

• ARMS OUT TO THE
SIDE USING POINTED
FINGERS.

WHILE STANDING – GIVE
YOUR DIRECTIONS TO
GO UP...
POINT YOUR FINGERS
TO THE FLOOR AND
GENTLY OPEN OUT
YOUR HANDS...
ROTATE YOUR HANDS
INTO THE ANATOMICAL
POSITION (PALMS TO
FACE FORWARD) –
DIRECTING OUT AND
AWAY FROM THE HAND.

NOW – ONE HAND AT A
TIME – SLOWLY TRACE
AN IMAGINARY LINE
ALONG THE FLOOR...
AND ON UP THE SIDE
OF THE WALL...

WITH THE HELP OF A
TEACHER – IMAGINE
RESTING YOUR ARM
(TO HELP IMPROVE
YOUR SENSE OF GOING
UP) , WHILE AT THE
SAME TIME POINTING
YOUR FINGERS OUT
TOWARDS THE WALL
(TO ASSIST YOUR
DIRECTIONS TO WIDEN).

THINK OF YOUR ARMS
GROWING FROM THE
MIDDLE OF YOUR
BACK (BETWEEN
YOUR SHOULDER
BLADES).

CAREFUL NOT TO LEAN
TO ONE SIDE, USE THE
OPPOSITE HEEL TO
DIRECT FROM

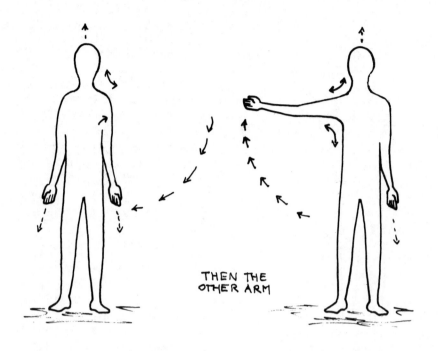

THEN THE
OTHER ARM

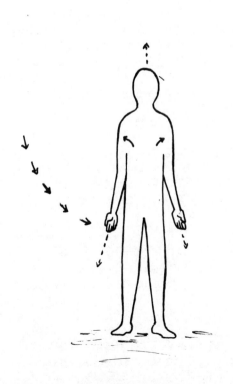

- ARMS OUT TO THE SIDE
(CONTINUED).

NOW — WHILE KEEPING THE
SENSE OF WIDENING AND
LENGTHENING — GRADUALLY
TRACE A LINE BACK DOWN
TO YOUR STARTING POINT
— AS IF FLOATING DOWN —

CONTINUE ON TO THE OTHER
SIDE, TRACING A LINE ALONG
THE FLOOR — UP THE WALL...
THEN, AS IF RESTING THERE,
DIRECT YOUR FINGERS AWAY
AND OUT OF THE HAND AND
ARM, ENCOURAGING YOURSELF
TO LENGTHEN AND WIDEN.

AGAIN — BRING YOUR ARM
BACK TO YOUR SIDE (AS
THOUGH IT WERE FLOATING).

DON'T FORGET TO DIRECT
UP (AND OUT, OR WIDE).

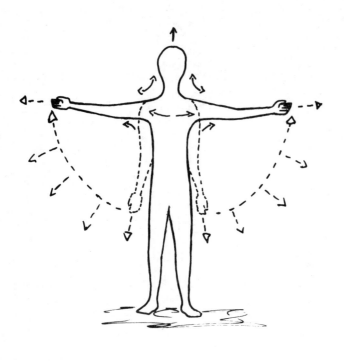

- ARMS OUT TO THE
  SIDE (CONTINUED).

PROCEED AS BEFORE
UP TO ROTATING YOUR
HANDS INTO THE
ANATOMICAL POSITION
(REMEMBER TO DO
THIS BY ROTATING
THE THUMB AROUND
THE LITTLE FINGER
AND NOT VICE VERSA).

THIS TIME TRACE A
LINE WITH BOTH
HANDS ALONG THE
FLOOR AND UP THE
WALL, UNTIL THEY
ARE OUTSTRETCHED
AND POINTING TO
OPPOSITE WALLS...

NOW REST YOUR ARMS
ON AN IMAGINARY
SUPPORT...

DIRECT YOUR FINGERS
AWAY AND OUT,
BRINGING THE ARMS
WITH THEM WHILE
WIDENING ACROSS
THE BACK AND THE
FRONT...

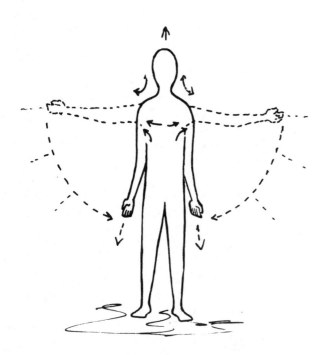

AND NOW, GRADUALLY
RETURN YOUR ARMS
TO THE SIDE AS IF
FLOATING DOWN ..

MAINTAINING THE NEW
DIRECTIONS OF
LENGTHENING UP
AND WIDENING OUT...

NOTICE HOW, WHEN BOTH ARMS ARE INVOLVED, YOUR WEIGHT
DOES NOT SHIFT OVER TO ONE SIDE OR THE OTHER, THUS
ALLOWING YOU TO DIRECT EVENLY OFF BOTH HEELS.

· ARMS TO THE FRONT (AND THE SHIFT OF BALANCE).

HANDS INTO ANATOMICAL POSITION... POINTING UP AND OUT TO THE SIDES. RAISE BOTH ARMS... ALLOW YOUR ARMS TO REST ON IMAGINARY SUPPORTS, AND THEN BRING BOTH HANDS SLOWLY FORWARD (BY POINTING), PAYING CLOSE ATTENTION TO THE CHANGE IN BALANCE...

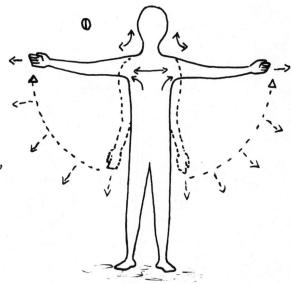

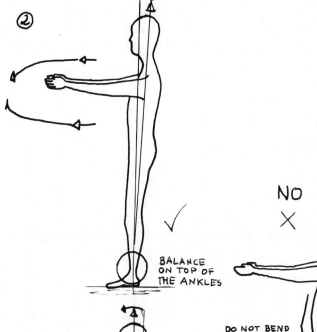

BALANCE ON TOP OF THE ANKLES

NO
×

DO NOT BEND AT THE WAIST

AS YOU BRING YOUR ARMS' WEIGHT TO THE FRONT — GENTLY COUNTERBALANCE BY PIVOTING BACK ON YOUR ANKLES...

BE VERY CAREFUL THAT YOU DO NOT USE YOUR TORSO ONLY — THEREBY PUSHING YOUR TUMMY FORWARD AND BENDING BACK AT THE WAIST AND HIPS.

YOUR ANKLES ARE THE PERFECT POINT ON WHICH TO PIVOT (KEEPING YOUR SPINE UNDISTORTED AND STILL CAPABLE OF LENGTHENING). DOUBLE CHECK WHILE WIDENING AND GOING UP — THAT YOU HAVE NOT PULLED THE SHOULDERS FORWARD EITHER. GRADUALLY RETURN YOUR ARMS TO THE SIDE (POINTING), PIVOTING ON YOUR ANKLES AS THE WEIGHT MOVES TO THE CENTRE.

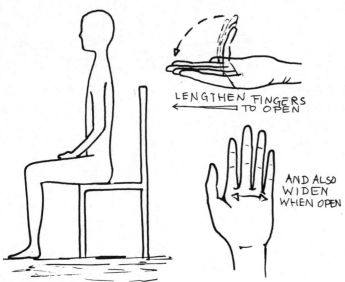

LENGTHEN FINGERS
TO OPEN

AND ALSO
WIDEN
WHEN OPEN

• ARMS (USING BACKS
OF HANDS TO POINT..)

NOW SEATED — USING
YOUR SITTING BONES
TO TAKE YOUR WEIGHT
AND PROVIDE A POINT
FROM WHICH YOU CAN
DIRECT (UP)——
HANDS RESTING ON
YOUR LEGS (PALMS
UP) — GRADUALLY
OPEN THE HANDS BY
USING THE EXTENSOR
MUSCLES, ALMOST
ROLLING OPEN, AND
LENGTHEN AND WIDEN.

NOW — THINK OF POINTING
WITH THE BACK OF THE
FINGERS — THEN, AFTER THE
TEACHER PLACES A HAND
OVER YOURS — GENTLY GUIDE
THE TEACHER'S HAND
OBLIQUELY TO THE FRONT
(AT TEN-MINUTES-TO FOR LEFT,
TEN-MINUTES-PAST FOR RIGHT)
AS THOUGH BOTH HANDS WERE
FLOATING...

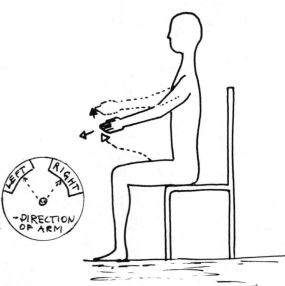

LEFT   RIGHT

— DIRECTION
OF ARM

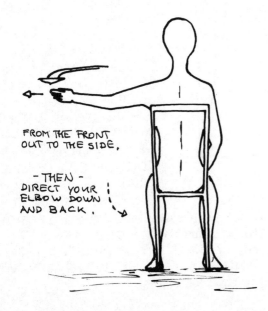

FROM THE FRONT
OUT TO THE SIDE,

— THEN —
DIRECT YOUR
ELBOW DOWN
AND BACK.

THEN USING THE BACK OF
YOUR HAND — SLOWLY
GUIDE THE TEACHER'S
HAND OUT TO THE SIDE...

NOW THINK OF DROPPING
YOUR ELBOW DOWN AND
BACK. WHILE YOU GUIDE
THE BACK OF YOUR HAND
TO THE RESTING POINT ON
YOUR LEG.

REPEAT ON THE OTHER
SIDE.

• USING THE BACK OF YOUR HANDS TO DIRECT OR POINT
AS A MEANS OF LIFTING YOUR ARMS TO THE SIDE.

① THE BASIC IDEA IS THE SAME AS BEFORE, EXCEPT
THIS TIME, INSTEAD OF POINTING WITH THE TIPS
OF THE FINGERS, LEAD WITH THE BACK OF THE HAND.
THIS CHANGE OF PERCEPTION AUTOMATICALLY BRINGS
A DIFFERENT SET OF MUSCLES INTO USE...

NOTICE THAT IF YOU THINK OF ONE HAND ONLY, THE OTHER
HAND WILL TEND TO DROP...

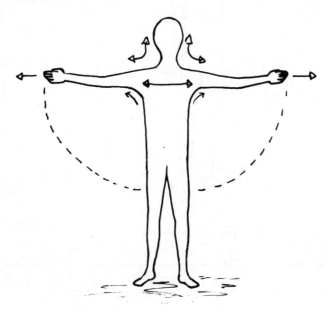

② WHILE LENGTHENING AND WIDENING, ALLOW YOUR
ARMS TO RETURN (ALMOST FLOATING) TO THE SIDE.
CONTINUE DIRECTING..

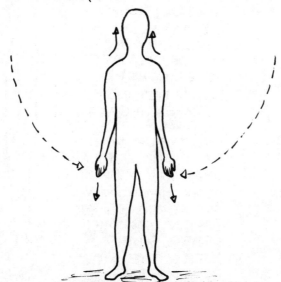

•RAISING YOUR ARMS/HANDS ABOVE YOUR HEAD,

BEGIN BY GIVING YOUR DIRECTIONS, STANDING ON
THE THREE POINTS OF EACH FOOT (LIKE THE STOOL)...

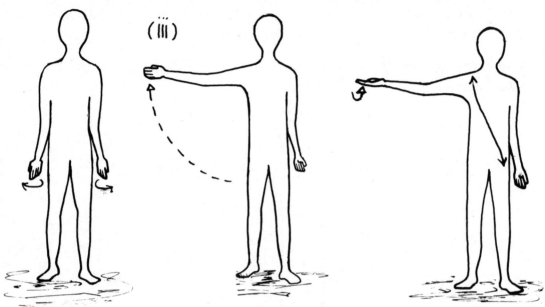

(ïïi)

ROTATE BOTH HANDS ON
THE AXIS OF THE
LITTLE FINGER (S)

TRACE A LINE ALONG
THE FLOOR AND UP
THE WALL TO THE
SIDE (EXTENDING)

ROTATE PALMS
UP, (ON SAME AXIS)
CONNECTING FROM
SHOULDER TO HIP

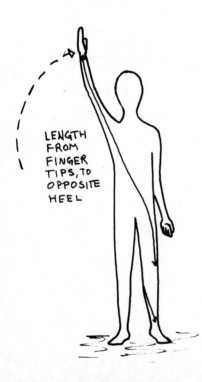

LENGTH
FROM
FINGER
TIPS, TO
OPPOSITE
HEEL

THEN CONTINUE THE
LINE UP THE WALL
AND ON TO THE
CEILING (USING
THE BACKS OF THE
HANDS/FINGERNAILS
AND-OR THE TIPS OF
THE FINGERS)...
LENGTHENING
BETWEEN THE HEEL
OF YOUR FOOT AND
THE TIP OF YOUR
FINGER......THEN
GRADUALLY BRING
YOUR HAND DOWN
TO THE SIDE...AND
REPEAT ON THE
OTHER SIDE.
NOTICE THE SHIFT
IN YOUR BALANCE.

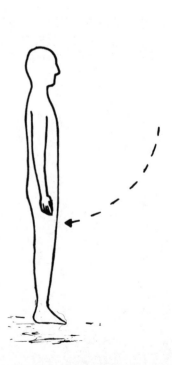

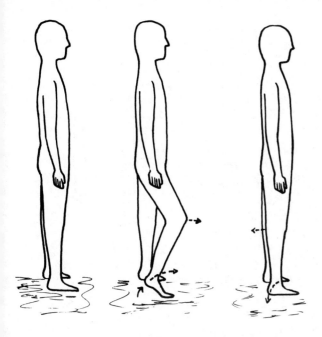

· WALKING.

GIVING YOUR DIRECTIONS TO GO UP AND WIDEN, CHECK THAT YOUR WEIGHT IS EVENLY DISTRIBUTED ON BOTH FEET, AND YOUR TOES ARE FREE... BEND YOUR KNEE FORWARD BRINGING YOUR HEEL OFF THE FLOOR AND YOUR WEIGHT ON TO THE BALL OF YOUR FOOT... CONTINUE DIRECTING FROM THAT PART OF THE FOOT... SEND YOUR HEEL TO THE FLOOR - STRAIGHTENING YOUR KNEE - CONTINUE DIRECTING...

DO NOT ALLOW YOUR HIPS TO TILT SIDEWAYS (PUSHED FROM THE FOOT), OTHERWISE YOU WILL NOT BE IN A POSITION TO DIRECT FROM THE GROUND THROUGH TO THE SPINE...

THE NEXT STAGE BEGINS IN THE SAME WAY AS BEFORE. FIRSTLY, YOU MAKE SURE THAT YOU ARE SUPPORTED BY THE GROUND WITH YOUR ANKLES, KNEES AND HIPS FREE

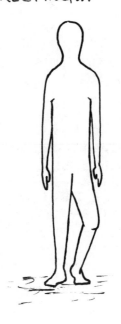

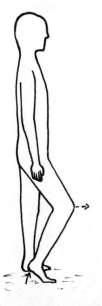

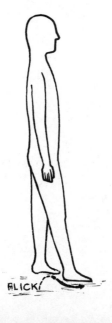

FLICK!

THEN – WITHOUT BENDING SIDEWAYS AT THE HIPS, BEND YOUR KNEE FORWARD AND BRING YOUR HEEL OFF THE FLOOR, DIRECTING FROM THE BALL OF YOUR FOOT...

NOW FLICK YOUR FOOT FORWARD TO WHERE YOUR TOES WERE (MORE OR LESS).

REPEAT ON THE OTHER SIDE.

· PREPARATION FOR WALKING

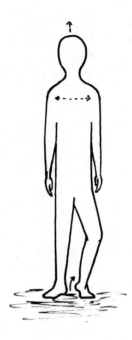

BEGIN WHILE STANDING AND
GOING UP IN THE FRONT AND
THE BACK, ALSO WIDENING...

MAINTAINING AN EVEN
DISTRIBUTION OF WEIGHT
ON BOTH FEET...
BEND YOUR KNEE FORWARD
LIFTING THAT HEEL OFF THE
FLOOR AND TRANSFERRING
THE WEIGHT (TAKEN BY THAT
FOOT) FORWARD ON TO THE
FRONT (BALL) OF THE FOOT...

THEN FLICK THAT FOOT OUT TO
THE SIDE WITHOUT DISTURBING
YOUR DIRECTIONS. (YOU WILL
SHIFT A LITTLE TO THAT SIDE
SIMPLY BECAUSE YOU HAVE
WIDENED YOUR STANCE)...

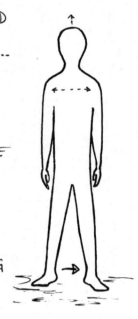

BEGIN AGAIN - THIS TIME ON THE OTHER SIDE, AND, LATER ON,
TRY IT WITHOUT GOING ON TO THE BALL OF YOUR FOOT.

AS BEFORE - WHILE STANDING (AND DIRECTING) - BEND YOUR
KNEE FORWARD, RAISING THAT HEEL
THEN - BEGIN USING YOUR OTHER HEEL TO DIRECT AWAY FROM (THIS
WILL BRING YOUR HEAD OVER THAT HEEL)...
LIFT YOUR FOOT OFF THE FLOO   MAKING SURE NOT TO
TILT SIDEWAYS AT THE HIPS OR WAIST, INSTEAD MOVE IN
ONE PIECE FROM YOUR ANKLE.

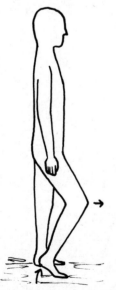
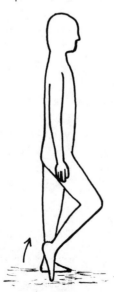
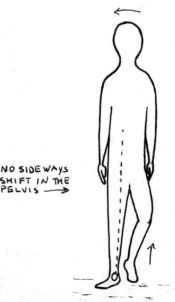

NO SIDEWAYS
SHIFT IN THE
PELVIS →

• WALKING (BACKWARDS).

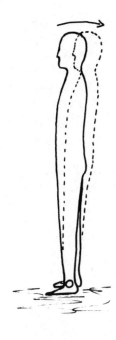

STANDING, AND
DIRECTING UP
AS WELL AS
WIDENING...
ALLOW YOUR
WEIGHT TO COME
BACK (ALL IN
ONE PIECE) OVER
YOUR ANKLES —
ALMOST FALLING.
DO NOT "DO" IT...
BUT GO WITH THE
NEED TO MOVE...

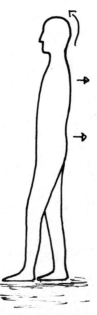

THEN IN THE
SAME MOVEMENT
BRING-OR FLICK
A FOOT BACK,
ACCOMMODATING
THE NEED FOR
SUPPORT...
CONTINUE TO
DIRECT, WHILE
WIDENING AT
THE SAME TIME...

REPEAT ON THE OTHER FOOT, AND THEN FOLLOW THROUGH
WITHOUT STOPPING THE ACTION, TO THE POINT WHERE YOU
ARE ACTUALLY WALKING BACKWARDS...
AS YOU GATHER MOMENTUM (WHILE MAINTAINING DIRECTIONS)
THE SWAY FROM SIDE TO SIDE WILL CORRESPONDINGLY BE
REDUCED, AND YOU WILL GRADUALLY MOVE IN A SMOOTHER
LINE — GOING UP IN FRONT, GOING UP IN THE BACK, AND
WIDENING ALL AT THE SAME TIME.

MAINTAINING THE "UP" AND REDUCING THE SWAY - - - - - - - →

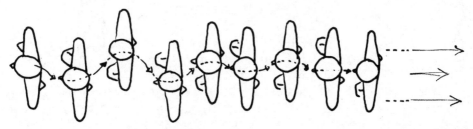

accelerando. - - - - - - - - -

THE REASON FOR PROCEEDING IN THIS WAY IS THAT WE
RARELY (IF EVER) WALK BACKWARDS, AND THEREFORE HAVE
FEWER HABITS TO AFFECT OUR DIRECTIONS. THIS ALLOWS US
UTILISE THESE EXPERIENCES WHEN WALKING FORWARD.

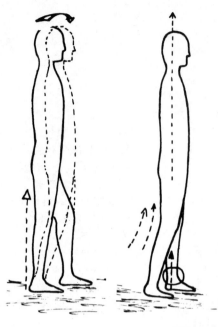

· WALKING (FORWARD).

BEGIN IN THE SAME WAY— AS FOR
WALKING BACKWARDS— BY TAKING
ONE STEP BACK ... AND THEN ....
FREE THE FORWARD LEG BY USING
THE BACK HEEL FOR DIRECTIONS...
NOW SHIFT YOUR WEIGHT OVER ON
TO THE FORWARD FOOT BY BRINGING
YOUR HEAD FORWARD AND UP OVER
THAT ANKLE...
NOW DIRECT OFF THE FORWARD
HEEL (NOT LIFTING THE BACK HEEL)
LENGTHENING AND WIDENING

DO NOT RUSH THINGS, INSTEAD
TAKE IT STEP BY STEP.....

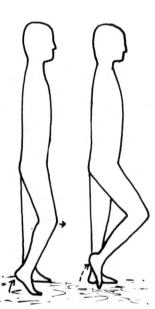

AT THIS STAGE YOU
CAN ALLOW THE BACK
KNEE TO BEND AND
BRING THAT HEEL
OFF THE GROUND...
DIRECTING WELL, UP
FROM THE FORWARD
HEEL , GENTLY LIFT
THE BACK FOOT OFF
THE FLOOR AND ,
SWINGING FROM THAT
KNEE , BRING YOUR
FOOT FORWARD TO
REST (HEEL FIRST)
NOT TAKING WEIGHT.
GIVING YOUR DIRECTIONS,
GENTLY BRING YOUR
HEAD FORWARD AND UP
OVER THE ANKLE/HEEL
OF THE FORWARD FOOT

CONTINUE IN THIS WAY UNTIL YOU ARE WALKING FORWARD ...
THE SWAY WILL BE MORE PRONOUNCED TO START WITH, BUT WILL
GRADUALLY DIMINISH AS YOUR MOMENTUM INCREASES.

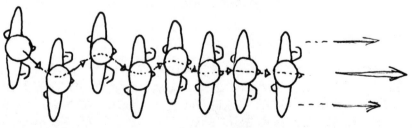

maintain the "up" Reducing the sway ---acceLerando......⟶

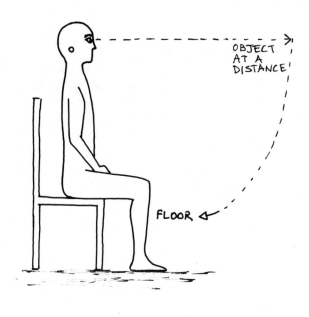

- EYES. AND THEIR FUNCTION IN THE MOVEMENT OF THE HEAD

WHILE SEATED, LOOK AHEAD AT A DISTANT OBJECT (DO NOT STARE) GRADUALLY—LOOKING ALONG THE GROUND— FOCUS ON OBJECTS NEARER AND NEARER TO YOU, UNTIL YOU ARE LOOKING AT THE GROUND IN FRONT OF YOUR FEET.

NOTICE HOW YOUR HEAD "NODS" OR PIVOTS FORWARD AS YOUR LINE OF FOCUS CHANGES. THIS IS THE FUNCTION OF THE ATLANTO-OCCIPITAL JOINT— (MANY PEOPLE PIVOT FROM THE SEVENTH CERVICAL VERTEBRA).

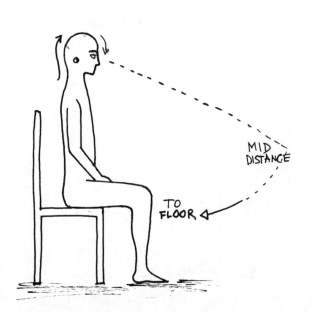

THERE ARE A NUMBER OF WAYS TO GO ABOUT THIS GAME,

① THE EYES MOVE FIRST— AND BRING THE HEAD IN TOW.
② THE EYES MOVE FIRST— THEN HOLD FOCUS (STOP) AND THEN THE HEAD NODS FORWARD. AGAIN THE EYES MOVE — STOP — HEAD NODS, ETC.. DO NOT STARE.
③ EYES AND HEAD MOVE TOGETHER (THE EYES A FRACTION IN ADVANCE OF THE HEAD).

IF YOU CANNOT (OR DO NOT) FOCUS, THEN YOUR SENSE OF AWARENESS IS NOT FULLY AT YOUR DISPOSAL. YOU MUST LOOK AND SEE.

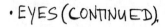

• EYES (CONTINUED).

AS BEFORE, LOOK
AHEAD AT AN
OBJECT SITUATED
ON THE SAME LEVEL
AS YOUR EYES —
GIVE YOUR
DIRECTIONS ...

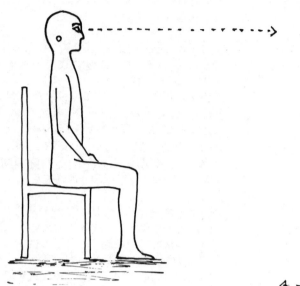

GRADUALLY BRING YOUR
FOCUS UPWARDS, AND
ALLOW YOUR HEAD TO
PIVOT AS YOU MOVE TO
LOOK ABOVE THE HEAD.
TAKING CARE NOT TO
PULL YOUR HEAD DOWN
INSTEAD OF FOLLOWING
THE EYES.

YOU CAN ALSO TRY
MOVING THE EYES
THEN THE HEAD —
THE EYES AGAIN,
AND SO ON, PAUSING
BETWEEN EACH TO
DIRECT.

THEN YOUR EYES
AND HEAD TOGETHER.

ALSO GO FROM
LOOKING TO THE FLOOR
AND BACK, THEN TO THE POINT ABOVE YOUR HEAD, ETC.

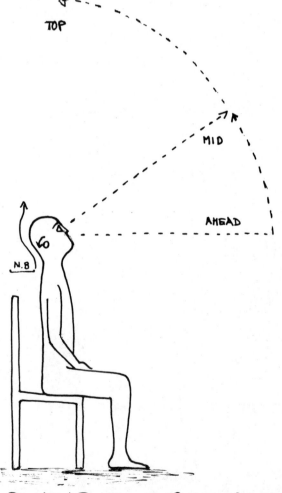

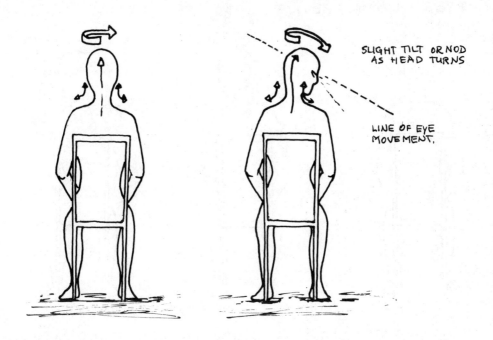

SLIGHT TILT OR NOD AS HEAD TURNS

LINE OF EYE MOVEMENT.

· EYES, AND THEIR EFFECT ON THE HEAD—NECK—BACK RELATIONSHIP.

SEATED THIS TIME, DIRECTING UP THE BACK, THE FRONT AND THE SIDES WHILE ALSO LOOKING AHEAD AT SOMETHING IN FRONT OF YOU (NOT PEERING AND PULLING YOUR HEAD OUT OF BALANCE TOWARD OBJECT)...
NOW THINK ABOUT LOOKING AT YOUR RIGHT SHOULDER, THEN SLOWLY TURN YOUR EYES (WITHOUT TURNING YOUR HEAD) TO LOOK IN THAT DIRECTION.---
THEN ALLOW YOUR HEAD TO FOLLOW...
NOTICE HOW FREEING THE NECK MUSCLES AND ALLOWING THE HEAD TO GO FORWARD AND UP (NOD) PROVIDES A MORE FLOWING ACTION, AND ALLOWS YOU TO SEE FURTHER...
RETURN TO CENTRE AND REPEAT ON THE OTHER SIDE.

NOW TURN THE EYES AND HEAD TOGETHER (TO EACH SIDE IN TURN).

NOTICE HOW MUCH THE EYES AFFECT THE MUSCLES THE NECK. IT REQUIRES CONSIDERABLE THOUGHT TO REDUCE THE HABIT OF TURNING YOUR HEAD WITHOUT LOO ING.

YOU CAN ALSO OBSERVE THE EFFECT OF LOOKING AHEAD WHILE TURNING YOUR HEAD SLOWLY FROM SIDE TO SIDE.

· EYES — USING THEM TO TURN.

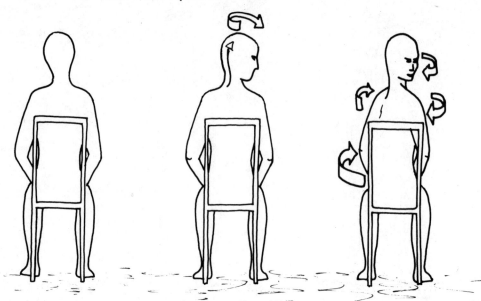

AGAIN SEATED — LOOKING AHEAD OF YOU, THEN MOVING YOUR EYES TO SEE YOUR RIGHT SHOULDER, AND THEN, ALLOWING YOUR HEAD TO TURN — CONTINUE TURNING SO THAT YOUR SPINE FOLLOWS (REFLEXLY) AND YOU ARE LOOKING BEHIND YOU (ASK YOURSELF; ARE YOU PUSHING WITH THE LEGS... OR SHOULDERS?) — THE CERVICAL AND LUMBAR AREAS ARE MORE FLEXIBLE THAN THE THORACIC AREA, AND THUS WILL ROTATE MORE. REPEAT ON OTHER SIDE...

NOW STANDING — REPEAT THE ABOVE — EYES FIRST — HEAD TO FOLLOW — THEN THE TORSO AND FINALLY THE LEGS.

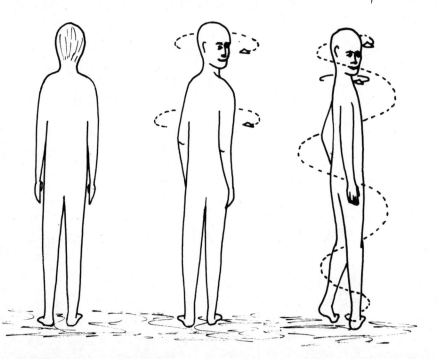

THE POSITIVE SUPPORTING REFLEX WILL KEEP THE RIGHT LEG AS A SUPPORT WHILE THE LEFT KNEE BENDS — LIFTING THE HEEL OFF THE FLOOR (BENDING AT THE TOES).

REPEAT ON OTHER SIDE.

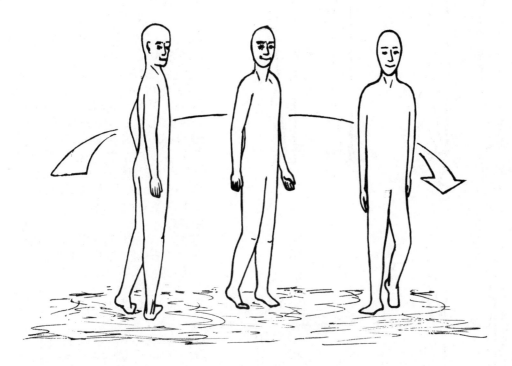

· USING YOUR EYES TO TURN WHILE WALKING.

HAVING LOOKED AT THE PREVIOUS GAME AND EXPERIENCED
THE EFFECT OF THE EYES ON THE HEAD-NECK-BACK
RELATIONSHIP, BEGIN WALKING WHILE LOOKING
AHEAD OF YOU (AS BEFORE)...
LOOK TO YOUR LEFT (OR RIGHT)...
ALLOW YOUR HEAD TO FOLLOW THE EYES, CAUSING
THE SPINE TO FOLLOW BY BENDING THE OPPOSITE
KNEE (AND ELBOW), THEN — AS YOU ARE MOVING — THAT
LEG WILL SWING AROUND TO SUPPORT THE TURN
NOW YOU ARE FACING FORWARD, AND-IF YOU CAN—
LOOK TO THE OTHER SIDE TO EFFECT A TURN ON
THAT SIDE...

NOTICE THAT ONE SIDE MAY BE EASIER THAN THE
OTHER...

ALSO OBSERVE THE GENTLE RELEASE OF THE STERNO-
MASTOID MUSCLES AS YOU COME OUT OF THE TURN.

THIS GAME IS AIMED AT ACTIVATING THE REFLEX TO TURN
BY USING YOUR EYES

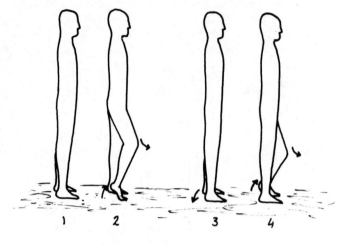

1 2 3 4

• MOVING LIMBS TOGETHER

BEGIN BY MOVING THE LOWER LIMBS....
WHILE STANDING —
INHIBIT AND DIRECT, THEN BEND ONE KNEE, BRINGING THAT HEEL OFF THE GROUND AND BENDING THE FOOT AT THE TOES, THEN SEND THAT HEEL TOWARDS THE GROUND STRAIGHTENING YOUR KNEE.
REPEAT THE PROCESS ON THE OTHER SIDE — THEN CONTINUE FROM SIDE TO SIDE IN ONE EVEN MOVEMENT.

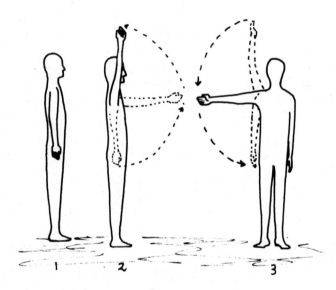

1 2 3

NOW THE UPPER LIMBS....
POINTING YOUR FINGERS TO THE GROUND, UNFOLD THE HAND USING YOUR AWARENESS OF THE BACKS OF THE HANDS TO DO SO, THEN DRAW AN IMAGINARY LINE ALONG THE GROUND AND UP THE WALL IN FRONT UP ABOVE YOUR HEAD — OUT TO THE SIDE AND BACK DOWN AGAIN.
REPEAT ON THE OTHER SIDE, UNTIL IT BECOMES ALL ONE MOVEMENT.

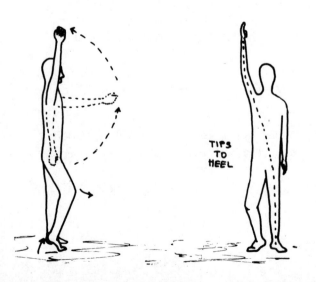

TIPS TO HEEL

FINALLY — SAME SIDE ARM AND LEG TOGETHER.
BEGIN WITH THE LEGS, AS BEFORE, AND WHEN IT IS FLOWING — INITIATE THE ARM MOVEMENT.
(THE ARM SHOULD BE UP WHEN THE SAME-SIDE HEEL IS UP)
ASK FOR LENGTH FROM RAISED FINGERTIPS TO OPPOSITE HEEL.

· SHOULDERS (BACK AND DOWN).

THE SHOULDER GIRDLE CONSISTS OF THE SCAPULA AT THE BACK, AND THE CLAVICLE AT THE FRONT, THEY MEET AT THE SIDE WHERE THE ARM IS ATTACHED(SUSPENDED). THE SHOULDER GIRDLE SITS LIKE A SADDLE ON TOP OF THE RIBCAGE, AND HELD IN POSITION BY MEANS OF VARIOUS MUSCULAR ATTACHMENTS FRONT AND BACK. IT IS FLOATING AND THEREFORE HIGHLY MOVABLE. IF YOU EXTEND YOUR ARMS OUT TO THE FRONT, YOUR SHOULDER BLADES WILL MOVE APART, AND OUT TO THE SIDES THEY WILL MOVE TOGETHER.

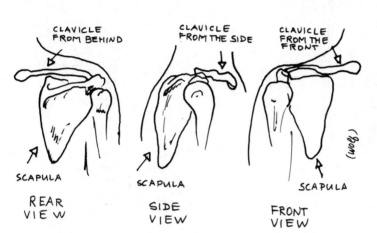

CLAVICLE FROM BEHIND

CLAVICLE FROM THE SIDE

CLAVICLE FROM THE FRONT

SCAPULA

SCAPULA

SCAPULA

REAR VIEW

SIDE VIEW

FRONT VIEW

(from)

· SHOULDERS BACK AND DOWN.

ALLOW YOUR HANDS TO OPEN BY POINTING TO THE FLOOR. THEN ROTATE THEM INTO THE ANATOMICAL POSITION (THUMB AROUND LITTLE FINGER). THEN–MAINTAINING DIRECTIONS– BEND AN ARM AT THE ELBOW (BY SENDING YOUR ELBOW BACK) SO THAT YOUR FINGERS ARE POINTING AHEAD OF YOU, AND FINALLY BRING YOUR HAND IN TO REST ON THE FRONT OF YOUR BODY– BY TURNING THE WRIST...
REPEAT THE PROCEDURE ON THE OTHER SIDE DIRECTING YOUR SHOULDERS BACK (AND DOWN–WITHOUT PULLING) BRING BOTH ARMS DOWN BY YOUR SIDE.

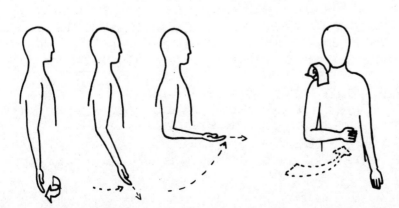

YOUR SHOULDER BLADES WILL BE CLOSER TOGETHER, AND YOU MAY FEEL AS THOUGH YOU ARE TIGHTENING, WHICH MAY NOT NECESSARILY BE THE CASE.

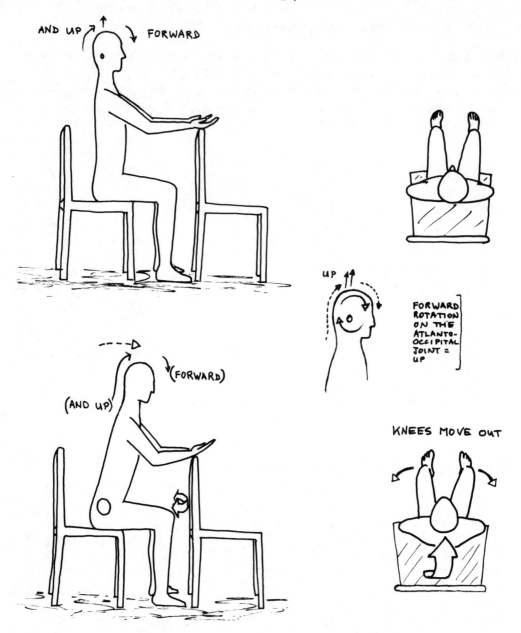

AND UP → ↑   ↘ FORWARD

UP ↑↑

FORWARD
ROTATION
ON THE
ATLANTO-
OCCIPITAL
JOINT =
UP

(FORWARD)

(AND UP)

KNEES MOVE OUT

· HANDS ON THE BACK OF A CHAIR (MOVING FROM THE HIPS)

SEATED - WITH THE BACK OF A CHAIR PLACED IN FRONT OF YOU -
POINT YOUR FINGERS TO THE FLOOR, THEN BEND AT THE ELBOWS
(BY SENDING THEM BACK) RAISING YOUR HAND IN THE PROCESS,
BRING BOTH HANDS TO REST (PALMS UP) ON THE BACK OF THE
CHAIR.
THEN - SENDING YOUR HEAD FORWARD AND UP - COME
FORWARD ON TO YOUR HANDS BY ALLOWING YOUR HEAD TO LEAD
THE MOVEMENT, WHILE KEEPING THE HIP JOINTS FREE.
IF YOUR HIPS ARE FREE AND YOU ARE NOT HOLDING WITH YOUR
LEG MUSCLES, YOUR KNEES WILL MOVE AWAY FROM EACH
OTHER AS YOU COME FORWARD.

• WHISPERED AH.

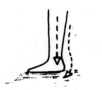

BEGIN BY ALLOWING YOUR WEIGHT TO
BALANCE OVER YOUR HEELS...
THEN— THINK OF IT SPREADING OUTWARDS
FROM THERE TOWARDS THE OUTSIDES
OF THE FEET...

NEXT— ALLOW YOUR HEAD TO
BALANCE FORWARD AND UP,
ABOVE THE HEELS, WHICH
HELPS PREVENT PULLING THE
STERNUM DOWN...
THEN— WHILE YOU DIRECT
THE HEAD FORWARD AND UP—
ALLOW YOUR BOTTOM TO DROP
BACK AND DOWN...

BOTH DIRECTIONS COMBINING
TO LENGTHEN THE BACK...

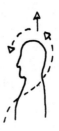 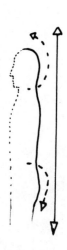

NOW— ALLOW THE SHOULDERS TO GO
(ROLL) BACK AND DOWN — ASSISTED BY
THE STERNUM LIFTING, AS THE HEAD
GOES FORWARD AND UP...
ALL RESULTING IN WIDENING ACROSS
THE CHEST AND SHOULDERS...

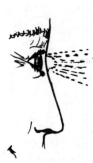

FINALLY— DO NOT
FORGET THE EYES,
AND HOW IMPORTANT
IT IS NOT TO STARE,
LOOK WITH INTEREST
AT AN OBJECT...

STARING MEANS THAT
YOU ARE LOOKING
FIXEDLY. AND THAT
IS WHAT TAKES
PLACE -- WE FIX, OR
TIGHTEN.

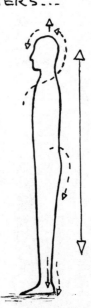

• WHISPERED AH (CONTINUED).

WHISPERED AH IS USED TO OBSERVE (AND CHANGE) EXCESSIVE
DOWNWARD MOVEMENT OF THE STERNUM (PULLING DOWN IN
FRONT), BUT WATCH YOU DO NOT PULL YOUR STERNUM UP EITHER.
USE IT ALSO AS A MEANS OF FREEING THE NECK FROM INSIDE,
AND BECOMING AWARE OF THE BREATHING (AND VOCAL) MECHANISM
AS A WHOLE _ IE., THE ENTIRE BODY...

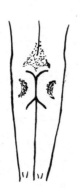

NOW _ WHILE STANDING
IN BALANCE _ MAKE
SURE THAT YOU ARE
NOT HOLDING OR
GRIPPING THE MUSCLES
IN YOUR BOTTOM...

INSTEAD _ ALLOW IT TO
DROP (TOWARDS YOUR
HEELS) AND SOFTEN,
THUS FREEING THE
LOWER BACK...

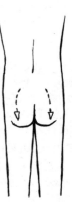

NEXT _ ALLOW YOUR TONGUE TO SOFTEN AND LIE ON THE FLOOR
OF YOUR MOUTH (SPREADING AND TOUCHING THE EDGES OF
THE LOWER TEETH)...
THEN _ ALLOW THIS FREEING OF THE TONGUE TO ENCOURAGE
YOUR JAW TO DROP (OR STOP TIGHTENING) AND AS A RESULT_TO
OPEN A GAP BETWEEN THE TOP AND BOTTOM TEETH _ ESPECIALLY
THE BACK TEETH...

AT THIS POINT _ WHILE BREATHING OUT
AND IN PASSIVELY (THROUGH THE
NOSE)_ THINK OF SOMETHING THAT
MAKES YOU SMILE...
THEN _ WITHOUT PREPARATION _ CHOOSE AN
OUT-BREATH, AND AT THE SAME TIME, PART
YOUR LIPS TO WHISPER THE WORD AH.....

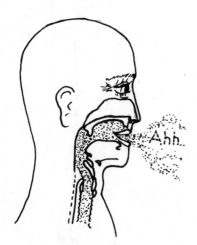

Ahh.

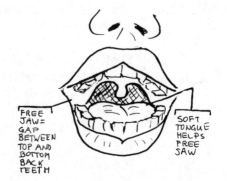

FREE
JAW =
GAP
BETWEEN
TOP AND
BOTTOM
BACK
TEETH

SOFT
TONGUE
HELPS
FREE
SAW

· WHISPERED AM. (CONTINUED).

THE MOVEMENT OF THE LOWER RIBS
(NUMBERS FIVE TO TEN) IS OFTEN
DESCRIBED AS BEING LIKE THAT
OF THE HANDLE OF A BUCKET,
SO THAT THE MORE WE BREATHE
OUT, THE MORE THE RIBS MOVE
INWARDS...
THE DIAPHRAGM IS SHAPED LIKE
A DOME, AND ITS MOVEMENT IS
LINKED TO THAT OF THE RIBS, SO
THAT AS THE RIBS MOVE INWARDS,
THE DIAPHRAGM MOVES UPWARDS
(SIMILAR TO THAT OF AN UMBRELLA).

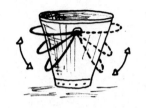

RIB MOVEMENT OUT TO
THE SIDES AND IN AGAIN

BREATHING OUT

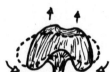

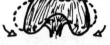

LOWER-RIB MOVEMENT   DIAPHRAGM'S MOVEMENT

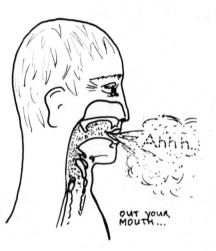

OUT YOUR
MOUTH...

NOW_ HAVING FOLLOWED THE INSTRUCTIONS IN THE PREVIOUS
GAMES - IMAGINE THAT YOU COULD TOUCH THE OBJECT YOU
ARE LOOKING AT (PREFERABLY ANOTHER PERSON).. AND_
BECAUSE IT IS VERY COMMON TO PULL THE TONGUE BACK INTO
THE THROAT - PLACE THE TIP OF THE TONGUE TO THE BACK OF
THE LOWER TEETH · AND WHISPER AM...

THEN_ ONCE YOU ARE HAPPY THAT
YOU HAVE EXPELLED AS MUCH
AIR AS YOU COULD WITHOUT
PULLING DOWN - ALLOW THE RIBS
TO SPRING OUTWARDS (SIDEWAYS),
AND THE DIAPHRAGM TO FOLLOW, BY
BECOMING FLATTER (AND LOWER),
AS THE AIR COMES IN THROUGH THE
NOSE.

BREATHING IN

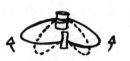

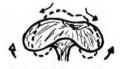

RIBS   DIAPHRAGM

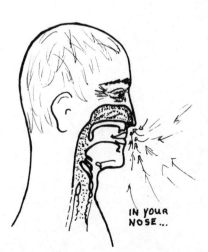

IN YOUR
NOSE...

SPIRALS

·SPIRALS (FRONT)

WHILE IN MONKEY (FOR EXAMPLE, STANDING AT THE PUPIL'S RIGHT HAND SIDE) PLACE YOUR RIGHT HAND ON POINT ①, AND YOUR LEFT HAND ON POINT ② ASKING FOR LENGTH BETWEEN THE TWO POINTS IN YOUR BODY WHILE LOOKING FOR THE SAME RESPONSE IN YOUR PUPIL.

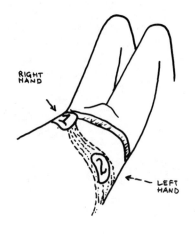

NOW PLACE YOUR RIGHT HAND ON ② AND THEN MOVE YOUR LEFT HAND TO POINT ③ (ON OR AROUND THE 7TH CERVICAL VERTEBRA) AGAIN - LENGTHEN BETWEEN THE POINTS

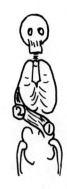

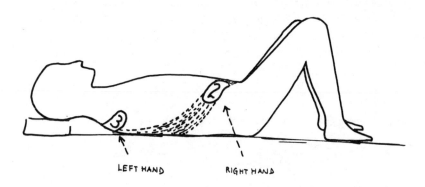

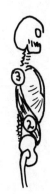

KEEPING YOUR LEFT HAND ON ③ CROSS OVER AND PLACE YOUR RIGHT HAND ON POINT ④. ONCE MORE ASKING FOR LENGTH .... FINALLY - LINK ④ UP WITH ① STANDING ON PUPIL'S LEFT.

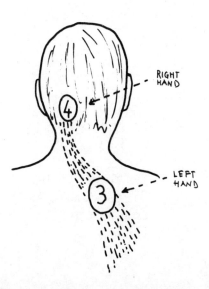

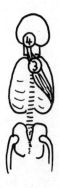

· SPIRALS (BACK)

ONCE AGAIN IN MONKEY ON THE PUPIL'S RIGHT SIDE, PLACE YOUR RIGHT HAND ON POINT ① UNDER THE PUPIL'S LEFT HIP AND YOUR LEFT HAND ON POINT ② UNDER THE ILIAC CREST — ASKING FOR LENGTH BETWEEN THE TWO POINTS...

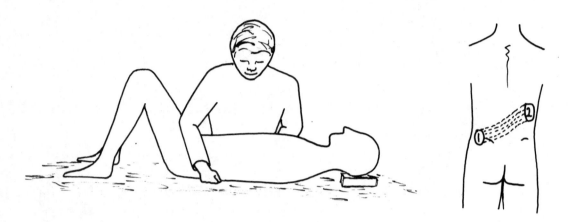

NOW CHANGE HANDS AND PLACE YOUR RIGHT HAND ON POINT ② AND MOVE YOUR LEFT HAND TO POINT ③ JUST UNDER THE RIGHT CLAVICLE AND AT THE RIGHT SIDE OF THE STERNUM ASKING FOR LENGTH BETWEEN THESE TWO POINTS...

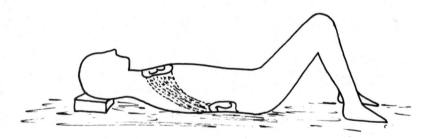

KEEPING YOUR LEFT HAND ON ③ IT WILL AGAIN BE NECESSARY TO CROSS OVER WITH THE RIGHT HAND AND PLACE IT ON ④ THE LEFT MASTOID BONE...

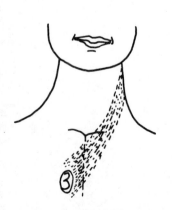

HAVING LOOKED FOR LENGTH BETWEEN THESE POINTS — CONNECT ④ UP WITH ①... YOU MAY NEED TO MOVE TO THE OTHER SIDE, AS BEFORE, TO DO THIS.

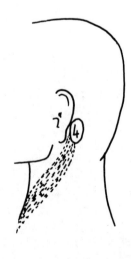

· SPIRALS (FRONT—LEG)

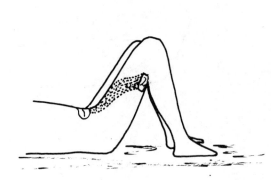

IN MONKEY AT THE
PUPIL'S RIGHT LEG—
PLACE YOUR LEFT HAND
ON POINT ① (AROUND THE
ILIAC CREST), AND YOUR
RIGHT HAND ON POINT ②
BETWEEN BICEPS FEMORIS
AND GASTROCNEMIUS...
OR ON THE KNEE ITSELF.)
THEN ASKING FOR LENGTH
BETWEEN THE TWO POINTS
IN YOURSELF AND, AS A
RESULT, IN YOUR PUPIL.

NOW CHANGE HANDS
AND PLACE YOUR LEFT
HAND ON POINT ② AND
YOUR RIGHT HAND ON
POINT ③ (THIS SIDE OF
ACHILLES TENDON AND
HEEL BONE)— AGAIN
ASK FOR LENGTH— IN
YOURSELF FIRST AND
THEN IN YOUR PUPIL.

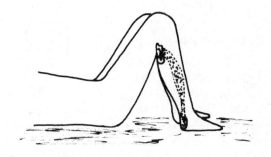

IF YOU CROSSED HANDS BETWEEN ② AND ③, YOUR LEFT HAND
WILL BE IN PLACE, OTHERWISE— PLACE YOUR LEFT HAND
ON ③ AND PLACE YOUR RIGHT HAND ON ④ (THE INSIDE
OF THE FOOT— BETWEEN THE BIG TOE AND FIRST METATARSAL)
AFTER LENGTHENING BETWEEN ③ AND ④ NOW LINK UP ①
AND ④

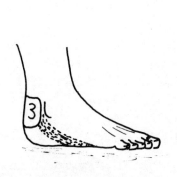
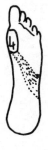
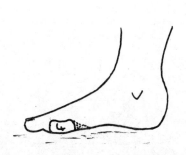

· SPIRALS (BACK — LEGS)

IN MONKEY—THIS
TIME ON THE
PUPIL'S LEFT,
PLACE YOUR
RIGHT HAND ON
POINT ① (BEHIND
THE RIGHT ILIAC
CREST) — AND
YOUR LEFT HAND
AROUND TO THE
INSIDE OF THE
BACK OF THE KNEE
POINT ②. THEN ASK
FOR LENGTH—AS
BEFORE— BEWEEN
THE TWO POINTS
IN YOURSELF, AND
SO, IN YOUR PUPIL...

THEN—KEEPING YOUR
LEFT HAND IN PLACE
MOVE YOUR RIGHT
HAND TO POINT ③
(INSIDE — BEHIND THE
ANKLE BONE). ONCE
AGAIN-LENGTHENING

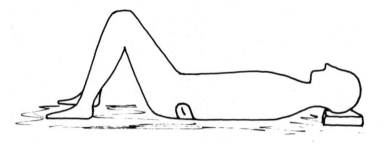

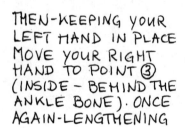

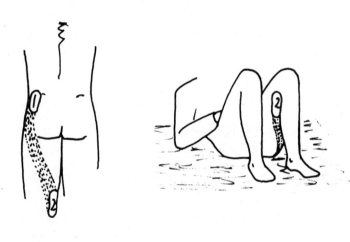

NOW— KEEPING YOUR RIGHT HAND ON
POINT ③— MOVE YOUR LEFT HAND TO
POINT ④ (OUTSIDE OF FOOT—BEHIND
THE LITTLE TOE). ASK FOR LENGTH
ONCE MORE AND FINALLY LINK UP
① AND ④.
· IN THE CASE OF FRONT AND BACK
SPIRALS, YOU CAN NOW LINK UP
POINTS ④ FOOT—WITH POINTS ④ HEAD.
· ALSO DON'T FORGET TO DO BOTH
LEFT AND RIGHT SPIRALS

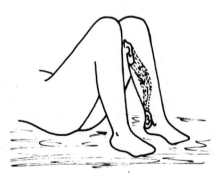

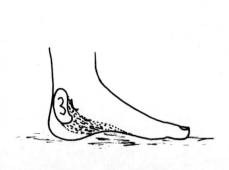

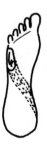

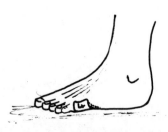

PART TWO

TERMS ONE TWO AND THREE COMBINED

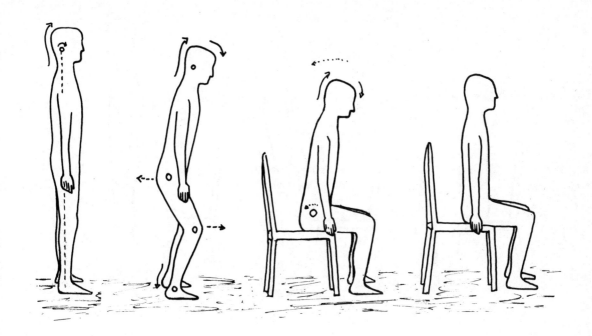

· SITTING (FROM STANDING).

IN THIS PROCEDURE WE NEED OUR ANKLE, KNEE, HIP AND
ATLANTO-OCCIPITAL JOINTS TO BE FREE, SO THAT WE USE
THE MINIMUM OF MUSCULAR EFFORT TO SIT DOWN, TO THIS
END, OUR PRIMARY CONCERN IS TO BALANCE THE HEAD ON
TOP OF THE SPINE (AND IN TURN, OVER THE ANKLES AND HEELS)
BY SUFFICIENTLY REDUCING NECK MUSCLE TENSION.

BALANCE EQUALS SUPPLENESS, WITHOUT WHICH OUR JOINTS
ARE COMPRESSED AND OUR MOVEMENTS STIFF.
SINCE MORE BODY WEIGHT IS DISTRIBUTED FORWARD OF THE
SPINE, ALLOW YOUR WEIGHT TO COME BACK OVER YOUR
HEELS AND MORE IN LINE WITH THE VERTICAL PLANE.
NOW YOU DO NOT NEED TO HOLD YOURSELF UP, WITH THE
RESULT THAT THERE WILL BE LESS COMPRESSION OF THE
JOINTS, INCLUDING THE DISCS, AND SINCE THE RIBS
ARE ATTACHED TO THE SPINE, WE CAN ALSO ALLOW FOR
FREER RIB MOVEMENT, AND THEREFORE FREER
BREATHING.

WITH YOUR HEAD GOING (ROCKING) FORWARD AND UP, YOU
ARE NOW IN A POSITION TO GO INTO THE CHAIR WHENEVER
YOU WISH. QUICKLY CHECK THAT THE ANKLES, KNEES,
HIPS, AND ATLANTO-OCCIPITAL JOINT ARE FREE, THEN,
AS IF YOU ARE GOING INTO MONKEY — HEAD AND KNEES
FORWARD, HIPS BACK, AND OFF YOU GO — CONTINUE TO
FREE THE NECK ETC., THROUGHOUT.

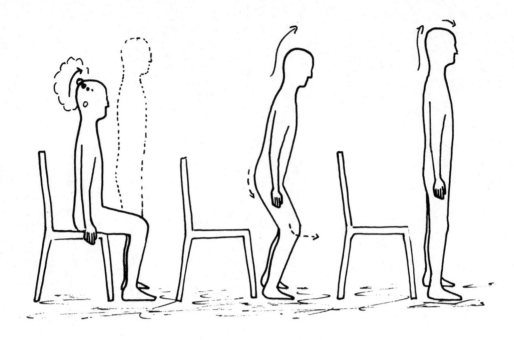

· STANDING UP .

SINCE THE GRAVITATIONAL PULL ACTS UPON EVERYTHING,
THE EFFORT NEEDED TO COUNTERACT IT WILL BE REDUCED
THE MORE BALANCE WE ACHIEVE; AND THE MORE BALANCE
WE ACHIEVE, THE LESS PULLING DOWN (SHORTENING AND
NARROWING IN STATURE) WILL TAKE PLACE, AND THE LESS
PULLING DOWN, THE MORE GOING UP (LENGTHENING. AND
WIDENING IN STATURE) WE CAN ACHIEVE.
CHECK THAT YOU ARE NOT FALLING FORWARD, BUT THAT YOUR
WEIGHT IS BALANCED OVER YOUR SITTING BONES AND IN
LINE WITH THE VERTICAL PLANE (CAREFUL NOT TO COME TOO
FAR BACK OR YOU WILL HAVE TO TIGHTEN YOUR LEG AND PELVIS
MUSCLES ETC.. UNDULY),
SO, ONCE SATISFIED WITH YOUR BALANCE, YOU ARE NO LONGER
GOING TO SAY "NO"... YOU ARE GOING TO SAY "YES" AND STAND

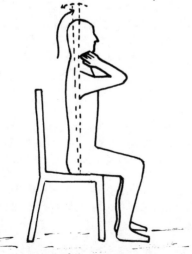

THIS IS A USEFUL WAY OF
CHECKING YOUR BALANCE
PRIOR TO AND DURING STANDING_
BRING YOUR FINGERS TO BEHIND
YOUR JAW AND UNDER YOUR
EARS (IN FRONT OF MASTOID)...
THIS WILL ADD TO THE FORWARD
WEIGHT, SO COME A LITTLE BIT
BACK ON TO YOUR SITTING BONES,
NOW ALLOW YOUR HEAD TO ACT AS
A BALANCER LEADING YOU
FORWARD AND UP_ AND RISE.

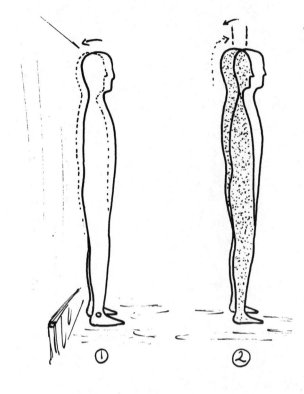

① ②

WEIGHT OVER
THE TOES.

ALLOW YOUR WEIGHT
TO BE LOCATED OVER
YOUR ------ HEELS

· THE USE OF THE WALL TO DEVELOP CONFIDENCE IN COMING BACK ON TO YOUR HEELS.

STAND WITH YOUR BACK TO THE WALL (BUT NOT TOUCHING) - WITH ENOUGH OF A GAP NOT TO RESTRICT MOVEMENT.

BECAUSE THE WALL IS THERE, YOU WILL BE LESS INCLINED TO WORRY ABOUT FALLING BACKWARDS AND THEREFORE CAN USE THE SITUATION TO CHECK YOUR BALANCE AND/OR POSSIBLE REACTIONS TO COMING BACK ON TO YOUR HEELS.

IF YOUR ANKLES ARE FREE YOU WILL BE ABLE TO INHIBIT LIFTING YOUR TOES KNOWING THAT THE WALL WILL STOP YOU FROM GOING TOO FAR BACK -
ONCE YOU ARE HAPPY WITH THE IDEA (AND THE EXPERIENCE) YOU CAN NOW USE YOUR HEAD TO NOD FORWARD AND ACT AS A COUNTERBALANCE BY FREEING YOUR NECK MUSCLES THAT BIT MORE.
FINALLY, ASK FOR A LITTLE MORE LENGTH (BACK AND FRONT) AND WIDTH.

{ F.M. (LATTERLY) DID NOT RECOMMEND RESTING YOUR BACK FLAT AGAINST THE WALL AND SLIDING DOWN }

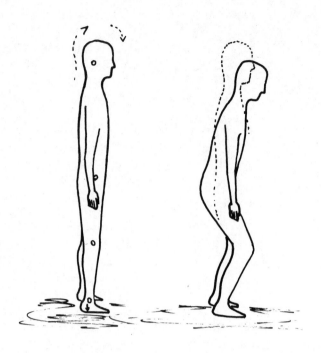

· MONKEY

AS BEFORE – WHAT WE ARE LOOKING
FOR IS BALANCE, BECAUSE WITHOUT
VERTICAL BALANCE WE WOULD HAVE TO
USE MORE MUSCULAR EFFORT TO PUSH OR
PULL SOMEHOW INTO MOVEMENT.
TAKE CARE NOT TO WANT TO DO IT – INSTEAD
BEGIN BY LOOKING FOR BALANCE WHILE
STANDING...
ALLOW YOUR WEIGHT TO REST OVER YOUR
HEELS, AND THE QUALITY OF CONTACT WITH
THE GROUND TO HELP FREE THE ANKLES...
ONCE YOU ARE HAPPY THAT YOU HAVE
FREED UP (AS BEST YOU CAN) THEN
THINK OF SENDING YOUR HEAD AND KNEES
FORWARD AND YOUR HIPS BACK....
AND GO INTO MONKEY.
AT THIS STAGE..IF YOU FEAR GETTING
IT WRONG – YOU WILL HESITATE AND
TIGHTEN: AND ONCE YOU DESTABILISE
YOUR BALANCE (BY TIGHTENING IN THE
ANKLES – KNEES AND HIPS) – GRAVITY
WILL SIMPLY AID BY PULLING YOU DOWN!
FORCES OTHER THAN MUSCULAR EFFORT
CAN BE USED IN CONJUNCTION WITH GRAVITY.

ONCE IN MONKEY, YOU CAN NOW GIVE A
GOOD IDEA OF UPWARD DIRECTION TO YOUR
PUPIL (SEATED OR STANDING).

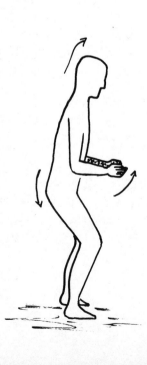

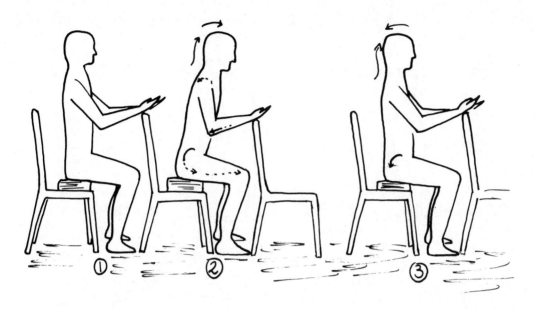

① ② ③

· ROCKING ON YOUR SITTING BONES (FREEING HIPS)

WHILE SEATED, BEGIN BY ALLOWING YOUR SITTING BONES
TO TAKE YOUR WEIGHT (THROUGH TO THE CHAIR)...
BRING YOUR HANDS UP TO REST (PALMS UP) ON THE
BACK OF A CHAIR PLACED IN FRONT OF YOU ...
THINK ABOUT FREEING YOUR NECK AND SENDING YOUR
HEAD FORWARD AND UP (AND YOUR KNEES FORWARD
AND YOUR HIPS BACK).
NOW ROCK GENTLY FORWARD ON TO YOUR HANDS —(IT IS
VERY EASY AT THIS POINT TO USE YOUR LEGS TO TAKE
THE WEIGHT, WHICH CAN BE BECAUSE YOU HAVE COME TOO
FAR FORWARD FOR YOUR HANDS TO SUPPORT THE
WEIGHT).
ONCE YOU ARE HAPPY WITH THE PROCEDURE THUS FAR
PULL TO THE ELBOWS AND WIDEN ACROSS THE UPPER
ARMS (SHOULDERS BACK AND DOWN ETC..).
NOW COME BACK INTO BALANCE ABOVE YOUR SITTING
BONES, AND REST YOUR HANDS ON YOUR LEGS.

Ⓐ IF YOU ARE NOT WELL ESTABLISHED ON YOUR SITTING
BONES—YOUR LEGS WILL PULL ON THE HIP JOINTS—
FORCING THE SPINE OUT OF SHAPE
Ⓑ IF, ON THE OTHER HAND, YOU USE YOUR SITTING BONES
FOR YOUR DIRECTIONS (UP) — YOUR LEGS CAN LENGTHEN
AND YOUR HIP JOINTS CAN BE FREED ETC..

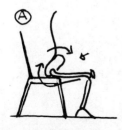

Ⓐ

YOU CAN END
UP SITTING
ON YOUR FEMUR

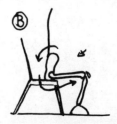

Ⓑ

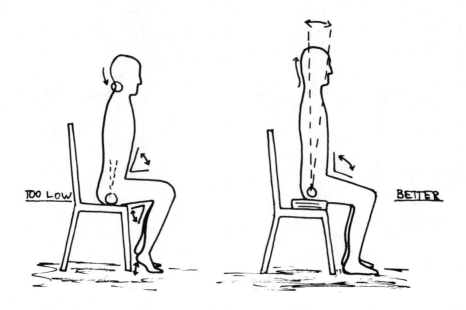

TOO LOW   BETTER

• CHAIR HEIGHT (PRE-WRITING).

NOTICE HOW IN THE PREVIOUS GAME THE CHAIR HEIGHT
APPEARS TO HAVE BEEN TOO LOW, NECESSITATING THE USE
OF TELEPHONE BOOKS (OR SOMETHING SIMILAR) TO HELP
RAISE THE SEAT (FOR PEOPLE WITH LONG HEEL-TO-KNEE DISTANCE).
IN ORDER TO COME FORWARD (FROM THE HIPS) OVER THE
WRITING SURFACE, WE NEED TO AVOID HAVING THE KNEES
HIGHER THAN THE HIPS, OTHERWISE WE WILL END UP
LIFTING OUR SITTING BONES AWAY FROM THE CHAIR (IF
NOT OFF THE CHAIR ALTOGETHER -- RESTING ON THE THIGHS)
PERHAPS EVEN TIGHTENING THE LEGS INTO THE PELVIS
AND LIFTING THE HEELS OFF THE GROUND — NOT TO MENTION
PULLING THE HEAD BACK.

BEFORE GOING ANY FURTHER - EXPERIMENT WITH THE
HEIGHT OF THE CHAIR (YOU NEED TO BE AT AN
ADVANTAGE WHEN IT COMES TO WRITING)
IF YOUR KNEES ARE HIGHER THAN (OR AT RIGHT ANGLES
TO) YOUR HIPS - THEN YOU ARE MOST LIKELY ON THE
RIGHT TRACK. WHILE SITTING NEAR THE EDGE OF THE
CHAIR CAN HELP ELIMINATE PRESSURE ON THE THIGHS, THE
SEATS OF SOME CHAIRS SLANT BACKWARDS, SO YOU MAY ALSO
NEED TO RAISE THE BACK LEGS TO CORRECT THE SLANT.

NOT →
GOOD

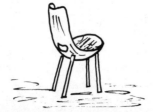

OTHER CHAIRS WILL PROVE
A WASTE OF TIME.....
FOR EXAMPLE THE "BUCKET"
OR PLASTIC "STACKING" CHAIR

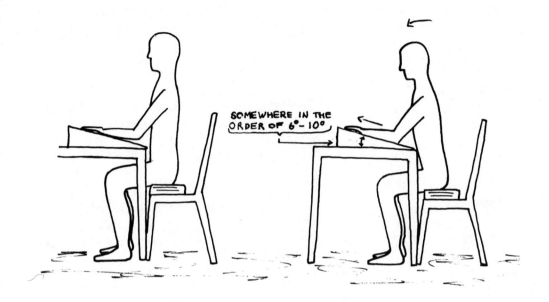

SOMEWHERE IN THE
ORDER OF 6° - 10°

· THE WRITING POSITION - BECOMING "THREE-FOOTED", AND
THE USE OF THE WRITING HAND

YOU WILL NEED TO SIT AS CLOSE TO THE DESK AS POSSIBLE
(WITHOUT PRESSING AGAINST IT). THIS, ALONG WITH THE USE
OF A WRITING SLOPE, REDUCES THE NEED TO COME TOO FAR
FORWARD FROM THE HIPS.

BRING THE NON-WRITING HAND UP TO REST ON THE SLOPE—
THEN COME GENTLY FORWARD ON YOUR SITTING BONES (IF
NECESSARY SLIDING YOUR ARM FORWARD)
ALLOW YOUR ELBOW AND FOREARM TO TAKE THE WEIGHT
AS THOUGH YOU WERE THREE-FOOTED (NOT UNLIKE CRAWLING).
KEEPING THE LENGTH FROM YOUR SITTING BONES AND THE
WIDTH ACROSS YOUR UPPER BACK AND CHEST, BRING YOUR
OTHER HAND UP TO REST ON THE WRITING SLOPE ...
NB.. KEEP A CLOSE WATCH ON THE WRITING HAND - IT IS
NOT UNLIKELY THAT YOU WILL TAKE SOME OF THE WEIGHT
AWAY FROM THE OTHER HAND (OR PRESS ON IT UNWITTINGLY)

POINT THE FINGERS OF YOUR WRITING HAND
AS IF YOU COULD TOUCH A DISTANT
OBJECT— THEN SLOWLY BRING
YOUR FINGERS OFF THE SURFACE
FOLLOWED BY THE REST OF YOUR
HAND — STILL POINTING .. EXTEND
AS FULLY AS IS COMFORTABLE—
THEN REST - CHECK DIRECTIONS.

· PREPARATION FOR USING A PEN ·

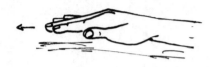

FOLLOW THE INSTRUCTIONS IN THE
PREVIOUS GAME ...
SUPPORTING YOUR WEIGHT AS IF
YOU WERE THREE-FOOTED, AND
POINTING THE FINGERS OF THE
WRITING HAND ....

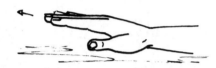

THIS TIME KEEP YOUR THUMB ON
THE WRITING SURFACE WHILE YOU
RAISE YOUR FINGERS (CONTINUE
POINTING) ......

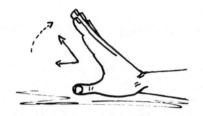

BECAUSE YOUR THUMB IS STILL
RESTING ON THE SURFACE ... YOU
WILL FIND YOUR WRIST WILL NOT
EXTEND TO THE SAME DEGREE AS
BEFORE .....

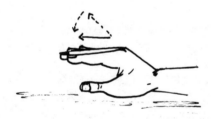

NOW - WHILE KEEPING THE WRIST
EXTENDED AND CONTINUING TO
POINT YOUR FINGERS ....
BRING YOUR FINGERS TOWARDS
YOUR THUMB (AND THE DESK),
DO NOT BRING YOUR THUMB UP TO
THE FINGERS .....

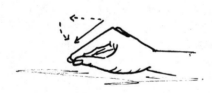

EVENTUALLY CONNECT YOUR
INDEX FINGER UP WITH YOUR
THUMB (CORTICAL OPPOSITION)

GO BACK TO YOUR DIRECTIONS AT
THIS POINT ..... AND THEN —

FLEX (BEND) YOUR INDEX FINGER AND THUMB BACK TOWARDS
THE HAND — THEN EXTEND THEM AGAIN — FLEX AGAIN, AND
EXTEND AGAIN .... REPEAT THE MOVEMENTS PAYING SPECIAL
ATTENTION TO THE EXTENSION (LIKE POINTING)

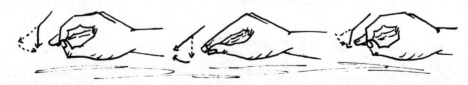

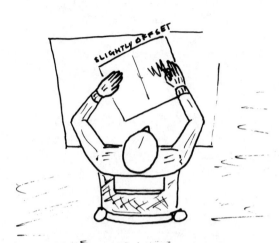

REPEATING THE INSTRUCTIONS WHILE
DRAWING THE PEN ACROSS THE PAGE

TO OPEN AND FREE THE
WRIST, CONTACT THE DESK
ON THE THUMB SIDE...

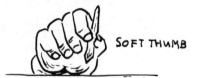

SOFT THUMB

· WRITING ·

HAVING FOLLOWED THE INSTRUCTIONS SO FAR, YOU WILL NO DOUBT BE AWARE OF THE IMPORTANCE OF MAINTAINING THE FREEDOM OF THE WRITING HAND, ARM AND SHOULDER .... SO, WITH THE WRITING PAPER PLACED IN FRONT OF YOU, USE YOUR SUPPORTING HAND TO STEADY IT AND KEEP IT SLIGHTLY OFFSET IF NECESSARY

TAKE THE PEN OR PENCIL IN YOUR HAND BETWEEN YOUR INDEX AND THUMB. USE THE MIDDLE FINGER IF NEEDED

THEN FLEXING AND EXTENDING YOUR FINGERS - MAKE UP-AND-DOWN STROKES ON THE PAGE.

THEN REPEAT AS YOU DRAW THE PEN ACROSS THE PAGE.

NOW MOVE YOUR WRIST FROM SIDE TO SIDE, DRAWING THE PEN HORIZONTALLY (USING ULNAR DEVIATION) —

FINALLY, TRY WRITING YOUR NAME.

POINTS TO WATCH : KEEP YOUR WRIST (HEEL OF THE HAND) IN CONTACT WITH THE PAGE (ALMOST ALL OF THE BASE OF YOUR THUMB AND THAT SIDE OF THE WRIST TOO). THIS MAY NOT BE AS EASY AS IT SOUNDS FOR SOME, BUT OBSERVE THE RELEASE IT BRINGS ABOUT IN THE ARM — SHOULDER AND NECK (NOT TO MENTION THE WRIST AND HAND). IT'S NOT A PROBLEM IF YOUR OTHER FINGERS NEED TO MOVE AS WELL AS THE INDEX AND THUMB .... CAREFUL YOU DON'T SHIFT OVER ON TO ONE SITTING BONE, FOR EXAMPLE, ON THE SUPPORT HAND'S SIDE, AND, AS YOU CONTINUE WRITING - WATCH YOU DON'T PULL DOWN IN FRONT — (VERY EASY WHEN IN THIS SITUATION).

· CRAWLING

SINCE OUR REFLEXES CAN EASILY BE INTERFERED WITH — WE NEED TO ALLOW PLENTY OF TIME SO THAT WE CAN MONITOR WHAT IS GOING ON, AND. IF POSSIBLE, TO BECOME AWARE OF THEIR EXISTENCE

HAVING COME ON TO YOUR HANDS AND KNEES — DIRECT YOUR HEAD AWAY FROM YOUR BOTTOM, AND YOUR BOTTOM AWAY FROM YOUR HEAD....

LOOK TO YOUR RIGHT HAND, AND — SENDING YOUR HEAD FORWARD AND UP (AWAY FROM YOUR BOTTOM) — GENTLY ROCK FORWARD .... JUST TO A POINT WHERE YOU BECOME AWARE OF A WISH TO SLIDE YOUR LEFT KNEE FORWARD....

THEN — HAVING BROUGHT YOUR LEFT LEG FORWARD (NOT TOO FAR) — ALLOW YOUR RIGHT HAND TO MOVE FORWARD TO UNDER YOUR RIGHT SHOULDER.

NOW LOOK TO YOUR LEFT HAND, AND ALLOW YOUR HEAD TO TURN (OR TO FOLLOW YOUR EYES). THEN CONTINUE.

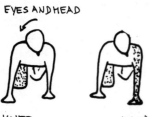

NOW ROCK GENTLY FORWARD AND BACK (THINK HEAD AND TAIL AWAY FROM EACHOTHER) — ALLOWING YOUR HIPS TO FREE AS BEST YOU CAN AND YOUR HEAD TO GO FORWARD AND OUT/UP

USING YOUR EYES — REFLEXLY MOVE INTO A CRAWL —

EYES AND HEAD   EYES AND HEAD   EYES AND HEAD

KNEE .... HAND   KNEE - HAND   KNEE ......   THEN HAND ETC..

EXERCISE CAUTION WHEN PREPARING TO CRAWL — BECAUSE, AS YOU COME FORWARD OVER YOUR HANDS, CONSIDERABLE DEMAND IS PLACED ON THE EXTENSORS OF THE WRISTS (AND HANDS)

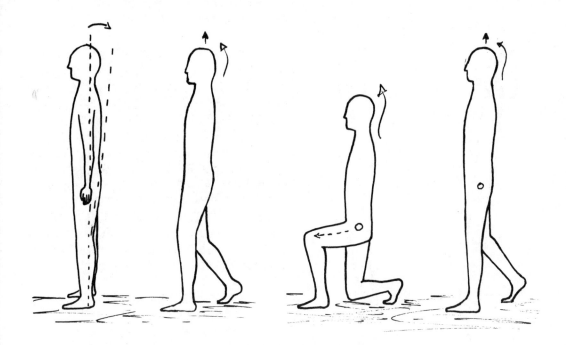

·TOUCHING THE GROUND ONE KNEE AT A TIME.

STANDING - ALLOW YOUR WEIGHT TO GO INTO THE GROUND,
THROUGH BOTH HEELS... GIVING YOU THE BALANCE NEEDED
TO FREE UPWARDS ...
PAYING CLOSE ATTENTION TO ALLOWING THE HIP JOINTS TO BE FREE,
TAKE ONE STEP BACK (ONTO BENT TOES).
THEN SEND YOUR OTHER KNEE FORWARD - BENDING IT WILL
BRING YOU INTO THE KNEELING POSITION (ON THE BACK LEG)
DO NOT WAIT AROUND - INSTEAD COME BACK INTO THE
UPRIGHT BEING CAREFUL NOT TO FIX IN ANY WAY...
NOW REPEAT THE PROCEDURE ON THE OTHER LEG.

DEVELOPING ON FROM THERE - AND HAVING GONE AS FAR AS -
GOING IN TO AND OUT OF KNEELING ON ONE SIDE - YOU NOW
SWING THE BACK FOOT FORWARD ...
THEN BRING YOUR WEIGHT FAR ENOUGH OVER ON TO THAT
FOOT-SO THAT YOU BEND YOUR BACK FOOT AT THE TOES...
CONTINUE INTO KNEELING BY SENDING YOUR FRONT KNEE
FORWARD (MAINTAINING AS BALANCED AN "UP" AS POSSIBLE)-
AGAIN, WITHOUT HESITATING, COME BACK INTO STANDING, AND
STRAIGHT AWAY ALLOW YOUR BACK FOOT TO SWING FORWARD.

FOLLOWING THE INSTRUCTIONS ABOVE - WALK FORWARD
TOUCHING EACH KNEE LIGHTLY TO THE GROUND AS EACH
STEP IS TAKEN (RIGHT FOOT STEPS AND LEFT KNEE TOUCHES, ETC..).
NEEDLESS TO SAY THAT THIS IS NOT A "MUSCLE PUMPING"
EXERCISE - BUT AN EXPERIMENT IN BALANCE.

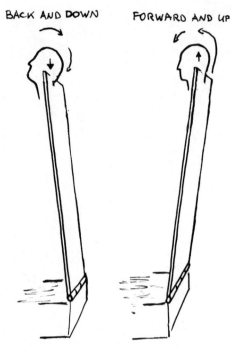

BACK AND DOWN   FORWARD AND UP

FORWARD ON TOES   BACK ON HEELS

• THE HEAD AS A BALANCER WALKING BACKWARDS.

IF WE ALLOW OUR ANKLES TO ACT AS THOUGH THEY WERE HINGES ON THE LID OF A BOX, AND OUR HEAD PLACED ON TOP OF THE LID TO ACT AS A BALANCER-SO THAT, WHEN THE LID WAS TOO FAR FORWARD, IT WOULD FORCE THE HEAD TO PULL BACK AND THEREBY STOP THE LID FROM FALLING ANY FURTHER .... ALSO IF THE LID WERE TO COME BACK — THEN THE HEAD WOULD NEED TO NOD, OR ROCK FORWARD TO REDRESS THE BALANCE

SINCE OUR TENDENCY IS USUALLY TO BE FORWARD ON OUR TOES... IT IS THEREFORE DESIRABLE THAT WE ENCOURAGE THE FORWARD BALANCE OF THE HEAD BY COMING BACK ON OUR HEELS.

THERE COMES A POINT WHERE YOU WILL BE TEMPTED TO LIFT YOUR TOES OFF THE GROUND.. INHIBIT THE WISH TO DO SO — AND WAIT FOR THE REFLEX TO BRING A FOOT BACK, HALTING THE BACKWARD FALL. HAVING FREE ANKLES AND THE HEAD GOING FORWARD AND UP WILL PROVIDE THE CONDITIONS FOR UNHINDERED REFLEXES.

NOW, WITH ONE FOOT BEHIND THE OTHER — DIRECT FROM YOUR HEEL TO YOUR FOREHEAD (ONE AT A TIME -- WITHOUT RUSHING)

THEN ALLOW THE MOMENTUM (AS YOU COME ON TO YOUR BACK HEEL) TO CARRY YOU THROUGH- AND THUS INSTIGATE A BACKWARDS WALK.

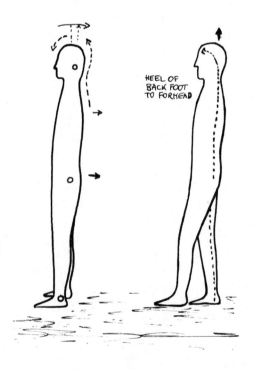

HEEL OF BACK FOOT TO FORHEAD

AS WE HAVE FEWER HABITS IN WALKING BACKWARDS...WE CAN DEVELOP OUR DIRECTIONS WHILE IN MOVEMENT.

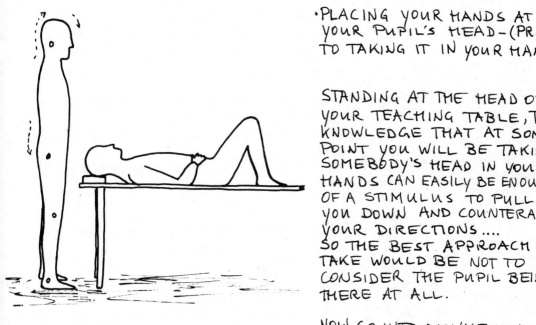

• PLACING YOUR HANDS AT
YOUR PUPIL'S HEAD — (PRIOR
TO TAKING IT IN YOUR HANDS)

STANDING AT THE HEAD OF
YOUR TEACHING TABLE, THE
KNOWLEDGE THAT AT SOME
POINT YOU WILL BE TAKING
SOMEBODY'S HEAD IN YOUR
HANDS CAN EASILY BE ENOUGH
OF A STIMULUS TO PULL
YOU DOWN AND COUNTERACT
YOUR DIRECTIONS ....
SO THE BEST APPROACH TO
TAKE WOULD BE NOT TO
CONSIDER THE PUPIL BEING
THERE AT ALL.

NOW GO INTO MONKEY IN THE
USUAL WAY BY PAYING CLOSE
ATTENTION TO YOUR HEAD –
NECK – BACK RELATIONSHIP
AND YOUR WEIGHT GOING THROUGH
THE HEELS INTO THE FLOOR.

ELBOW
BACK

HAND
UP

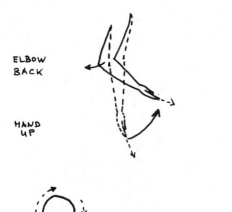

NOW — POINTING YOUR FINGERS
TO THE FLOOR – SEND YOUR
ELBOWS BACK AND BRING
YOUR HANDS UP TO REST
ON THE TABLE (EITHER SIDE
OF THE PUPIL'S HEAD).

SENDING YOUR KNEES
FORWARD, GENTLY BRING
YOUR WEIGHT OVER ON TO
YOUR HANDS AS IF YOU
WERE FOUR-FOOTED ....
TAKE CARE AT THIS STAGE
NOT TO PULL DOWN OR FIX.

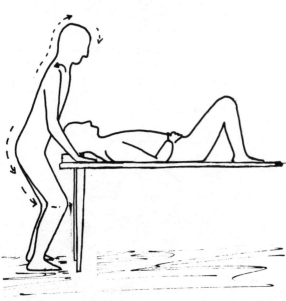

REMEMBERING YOUR HEELS,
DIRECT YOUR SHOULDERS
BACK AND DOWN (AS IF
YOUR SPINE WAS ADVANCING
BETWEEN THE SHOULDERS)
WIDEN ACROSS THE UPPER
BACK, ARMS AND CHEST.
OBSERVE YOUR BREATHING.

·TAKING THE PUPIL'S HEAD.

GO BACK OVER THE PREVIOUS SET OF INSTRUCTIONS, UP TO
WHERE YOU PLACE YOUR HANDS ON EITHER SIDE OF THE
PUPIL'S HEAD...

THEN TAKE ONE HAND OFF THE TABLE_(BECOMING
THREE-FOOTED AS YOU DO SO)_ AND PLACE IT UNDER
THE PUPIL'S HEAD (PALM FACING UP - JUST BEHIND THE
EAR)
NOW BRING YOUR OTHER HAND UP TO REST_IN THE SAME
WAY- BEHIND THE OTHER EAR.

HAVING ARRIVED AT THIS POINT_
TAKE A MOMENT TO CHECK YOUR
DIRECTIONS

NOW TURN THE PUPIL'S HEAD TO
THE LEFT (OR ASK YOUR PUPIL
TO TURN IT FOR YOU -- USING THE
EYES FIRST TO LOOK TO THAT SIDE)
AND MOVE YOUR RIGHT HAND UNDER.
THEN REPEAT THE PROCEDURE ON
THE OTHER SIDE.

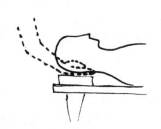

HEAD TURNED TO THE LEFT
AND YOUR RIGHT HAND IS
POSITIONED AT THE BACK

LEFT HAND POSITIONED

FINALLY - WITH YOUR TWO
HANDS NOW WELL PLACED
TO DIRECT - BRING THE
HEAD TO REST FACING
UPWARDS...
NOW LEAVE YOUR HANDS
ALONE -WITH AS LITTLE
"DOING" IN THEM AS YOU
CAN POSSIBLY MANAGE
(RELEASING YOUR NECK AND
THIGH MUSCLES).

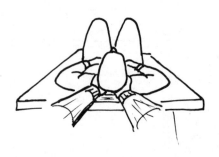

COME TO REST

·BOOK HEIGHT, (AND TAKING PUPIL'S HEAD).

TO DISCOVER AN APPROPRIATE BOOK HEIGHT FOR YOUR PUPIL,
FOLLOW THE PREVIOUS INSTRUCTIONS UP TO WHERE YOU HAVE
YOUR PUPIL'S HEAD IN BOTH HANDS...
THEN- HAVING PAUSED FOR A MOMENT TO CHECK YOUR OWN
DIRECTIONS - TURN THE HEAD SLIGHTLY INTO ONE HAND, AND
REMOVE THE BOOKS WITH YOUR OTHER HAND...
THEN PLACE YOUR FREE HAND UNDER THE OTHER SIDE OF
THE PUPIL'S HEAD...
NOW- NOT FORGETTING YOUR OWN DIRECTIONS OF HEAD
FORWARD AND UP, PULLING TO THE ELBOWS, FREE ANKLES,
KNEES AND HIPS ETC.. GRADUALLY LOWER YOUR PUPIL'S
HEAD UNTIL A SENSE OF ELASTIC, FILLING OUT, OR "GIVE" IS
PERCEIVED IN THE PUPIL...
THEN- GENTLY TURN THE HEAD INTO ONE HAND ONCE AGAIN,
AND REPLACE THE BOOKS WITH YOUR FREE HAND TO AS
CLOSE TO THE DISCOVERED HEIGHT AS POSSIBLE. N.B. IT IS
BETTER TO HAVE TOO MANY BOOKS THAN TOO FEW.

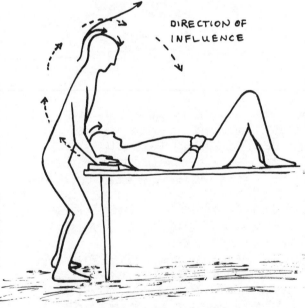

DIRECTION OF
INFLUENCE

BEFORE REMOVING OUR
HANDS, WE NEED THEM TO BE
AS FREE OF "DOING" AS WE
CAN POSSIBLY MANAGE.
THEREBY PROVIDING AN
ENCOURAGING STIMULUS FOR
THE PUPIL TO INHIBIT NECK
MUSCLE TENSION, AND
DIRECT THE HEAD FORWARD
AND UP...

IN ALL CREATURES, THE HEAD
LEADS AND THE BODY
FOLLOWS. OUR DIRECTIONS
HELP ENCOURAGE THIS IN
THE PUPIL.

WHEN LYING IN SEMI-SUPINE
THE IDEA IS NOT TO "RELAX"
OR FALL ASLEEP, IT IS TO
WORK ON AND DEVELOP
INHIBITION, THUS CLEARING
THE WAY FOR DIRECTION.
THE STUDENTS AT F.M.'s
SCHOOL CALLED IT
"INHIBITION WORK".

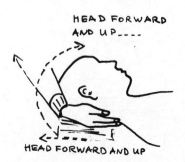

HEAD FORWARD
AND UP....

HEAD FORWARD AND UP

• TAKING A LEG OUT TO THE SIDE - FREEING THE HIPS AND ENCOURAGING LENGTH.

WITH YOUR PUPIL IN SEMI-SUPINE, LOCATE THE HAMSTRINGS (BEHIND THE KNEE) BY POSITIONING YOUR LEFT HAND ON THE INSIDE OF THE LEFT KNEE.. WITH YOUR FINGERS TUCKED IN BEHIND THE BENT KNEE _ AND YOUR RIGHT HAND ON THE OUTSIDE WITH THE FINGERS ALSO IN UNDER THE KNEE...
WHEN YOU HAVE CONTACTED THE TENDONS (TWO ON THE INSIDE AND ONE ON THE OUTSIDE OF THE LEG)... REST FOR A MOMENT TO SETTLE YOUR HANDS AND CHECK OVER YOUR DIRECTIONS ...

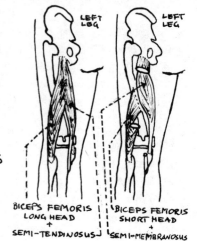

LEFT LEG   LEFT LEG

BICEPS FEMORIS LONG HEAD + SEMI-TENDINOSUS | BICEPS FEMORIS SHORT HEAD + SEMI-MEMBRANOSUS

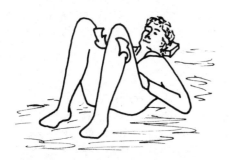

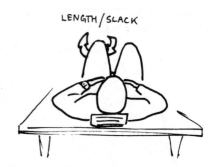

LENGTH/SLACK

BECAUSE WE TEND TO SHORTEN THE HAMSTRINGS ON THE INSIDE OF THE LEG -- WE WILL BE LOOKING TO GIVE SOME "SLACK" TO THAT PART WHILE LENGTHENING THE OUTSIDE..
IN ORDER TO ACHIEVE THIS, WE NEED TO DIRECT OUR LEFT HAND TOWARDS THE PUPIL AND OUR RIGHT HAND TOWARDS OURSELVES
NOW_THINKING ABOUT THE DIRECTION IN WHICH THE BACK SPIRAL COMES AROUND TO THE FRONT OF THE LEG _ AND EFFECTIVELY FEEDS IN TO YOUR LEFT HAND ---
GENTLY GUIDE THE LEG OUT TO THE SIDE _ STOPPING AS SOON AS YOU DETECT THE SLIGHTEST RESISTANCE _ OR AS SOON AS YOU NOTICE THE INSIDE OF THE FOOT LIFTING OFF THE SURFACE OF THE TABLE. _ NOW REPEAT ON OTHER LEG...

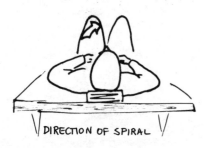

DIRECTION OF SPIRAL

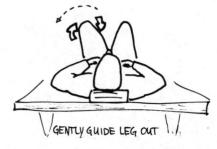

GENTLY GUIDE LEG OUT

• LIFTING THE PUPIL'S LEG — AND
DEVELOPING INHIBITION.

BECAUSE THE PUPIL MAY
FIND IT DIFFICULT NOT TO
HELP YOU WHEN MOVING THE
LEG — IT CAN SOMETIMES BE
A GOOD IDEA TO ASK HIM/HER
TO THINK OF THE OTHER LEG
OR ANOTHER PART OF THE
BODY ALTOGETHER — BUT
OF COURSE, IF THIS DOES
NOT WORK, IT WOULD BE TOO
SOON TO PROCEED FURTHER
THAN SIMPLY TAKING SOME
OF THE WEIGHT OFF THE
FOOT..

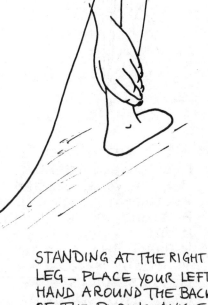

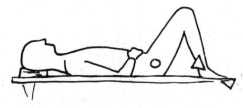

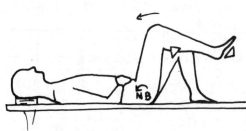

STANDING AT THE RIGHT
LEG — PLACE YOUR LEFT
HAND AROUND THE BACK
OF THE PUPIL'S ANKLE
(WITH YOUR THUMB TO
THE INSIDE)..
THEN GENTLY LIFT THE
FOOT — PLACING YOUR
RIGHT HAND UNDERNEATH

NOW — THINKING OF WHERE
THE LEG MOVES AT THE
HIP JOINT — RAISE THE LEG
AND MOVE YOUR LEFT
HAND UP TO THE MIDDLE
OF GASTROCNEMIUS (THE
CALF MUSCLE)...

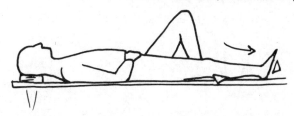

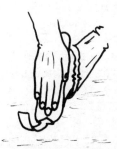

AND LOWER THE LEG SLOWLY —
KEEPING IN MIND THAT ONLY WITH
A VERY FREE LOWER BACK
SHOULD YOU STRAIGHTEN
THE LEG. ONCE IT IS LOWERED,
PRESSURE APPLIED TO THE
HEEL CAN HELP TO MOVE THE
FOOT AT THE ANKLE.

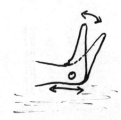

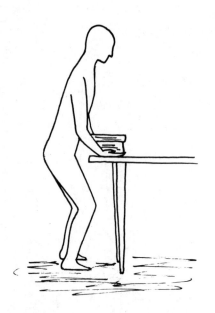

• LIFTING A WEIGHT.

BEGIN BY GOING INTO MONKEY AT
THE HEAD OF YOUR TEACHING TABLE.
THEN OPEN YOUR HANDS OUT BY
POINTING YOUR FINGERS TO THE
FLOOR - - -
NOW BRING BOTH HANDS UP TO REST
(PALMS UP) ON THE TABLE, AND USE
THE IDEA OF BEING FOUR-FOOTED TO
DIRECT YOUR SHOULDERS BACK
AND DOWN (INTO YOUR BACK) ..
NOW HAVE SOMEONE PLACE WEIGHT
ON YOUR HANDS (IN THIS CASE
TELEPHONE BOOKS WERE USED)...

AVOID "GETTING READY"..SINCE THE
MOST LIKELY RESULT IS TIGHTEN-
ING OF YOUR BICEPS AND
PECTORALS, SO EXCLUDING ANY OTHER
POSSIBILITIES, OR ALTERNATIVES TO
HABIT...
WITHOUT CHANGING THE RELATIVE
POSITION OF YOUR SHOULDERS,
ELBOWS, WRISTS AND HANDS.
COME INTO STANDING, BRINGING
THE BOOKS WITH YOU -(NOT
FORGETTING TO SEND YOUR KNEES
FORWARD AS A PRELIMINARY TO
MOVING), DIRECTING AS YOU GO.

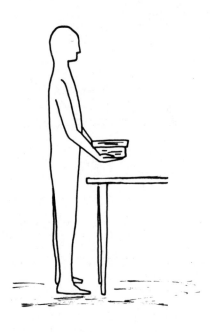

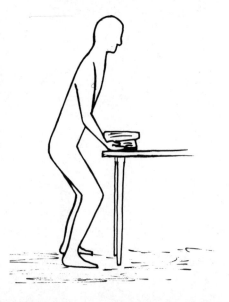

ONCE STANDING — ALLOW THE
WEIGHT TO GO THROUGH YOUR
HEELS -- WHILE AT THE SAME
TIME OBSERVING HOW THE BACK
MUSCLES ARE INVOLVED.

THE NEXT STEP IS SIMPLY TO
REPLACE THE BOOKS ON THE
TABLE BY GOING INTO MONKEY
ONCE MORE (OBSERVING YOUR
BALANCE AS YOU GO) .

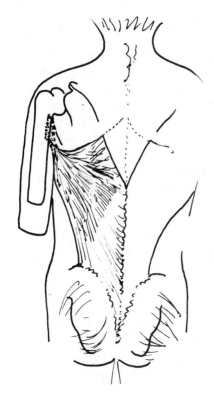

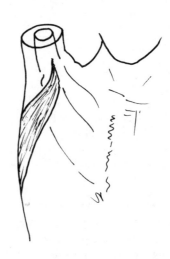

• SHOULDER WORK — AND THE MECHANISM OF CONTRACTION —

NARROWING ACROSS THE UPPER ARMS AND CHEST IS INFLUENCED LARGELY BY LATISSIMUS DORSI AND PECTORALIS MAJOR PULLING THE ARMS INWARDS.

LATISSIMUS DORSI'S ORIGIN IS FROM HALF WAY DOWN THE THORACIC SPINE (T.6.)—ALL THE WAY DOWN TO THE SACRUM — IT THEN COMES AROUND THE SIDE AND INSERTS INTO THE UPPER ARM BONE (HUMERUS).

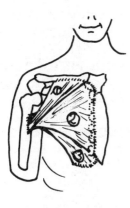

PECTORALIS MAJOR IS MADE UP OF THREE SECTIONS
① THE CLAVICULAR PORTION — ITS ORIGIN BEING MUCH OF THE CLAVICLE,
② THE STERNO COSTAL PORTION — ITS ORIGIN BEING THE STERNUM AND RIBS,
③ THE ABDOMINAL FASCICULI — WITH ITS ORIGIN BEING PART OF THE APONEUROSIS OF THE ABDOMEN'S EXTERNAL OBLIQUE MUSCLES.
ALL THREE INSERT INTO THE UPPER ARM NEAR LATISSIMUS DORSI.

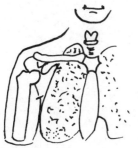

CONTRACTION WILL ALSO AFFECT THE LUNGS

WITHOUT YOUR WIDENING ACROSS THE UPPER ARM AND CHEST, IT IS MORE DIFFICULT TO ACHIEVE IT IN YOUR PUPIL.

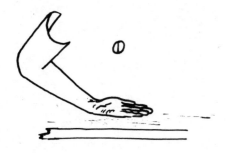

·RELEASING YOUR PUPIL'S SHOULDER

BEGIN BY GOING INTO MONKEY AT THE SIDE OF THE TABLE (BESIDE THE PUPIL'S RIGHT SHOULDER..) NOW—POINTING YOUR FINGERS TO THE FLOOR—BRING YOUR LEFT HAND UP TO REST ON THE TABLE (JUST BEHIND THE SHOULDER).. AND THEN—KEEPING YOUR WIDTH—SLIDE YOUR HAND UNDER...

TAKE CARE NOT TO PUSH AGAINST THE SHOULDER BLADE, AND CAUSE A POSSIBLE REACTION...

NOW BRING YOUR RIGHT HAND UP TO REST ON THE PECTORALS—WITH YOUR THUMB POINTING INTO THE ARMPIT (AT THE INSERTION OF L. DORSI).

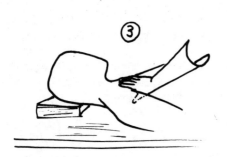

ASKING YOUR PUPIL TO REST THE SHOULDER ON YOUR HAND

YOU MAY FIND THAT THE SHOULDER IS RAISED QUITE HIGH OFF THE TABLE—IF THIS IS THE CASE... DO NOT FORCE IT DOWN—(YOUR HAND IS THERE ONLY TO GIVE ENCOURAGEMENT WITH DIRECTION) INSTEAD.. SIMPLY BRING YOUR LEFT HAND UP TO MEET THE BACK OF THE SHOULDER, AND DIRECT BOTH HANDS INTO EACH OTHER ... NOW COME A LITTLE MORE ON TO YOUR HEELS AND WAIT FOR A CHANGE TO APPEAR...

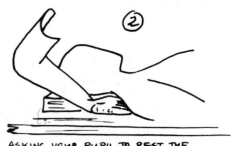

WHEN YOU OBSERVE AN "ELASTIC GIVE"—SLIDE YOUR LEFT HAND SIDEWAYS AND GENTLY OUT... THEN COME INTO STANDING.

IF YOU WISH TO LIFT THE SHOULDER TO SLIP YOUR LEFT HAND LOWER ON TO THE SCAPULA—USE YOUR RIGHT HAND UNDER THE ARM AND THE SHOULDER BLADE TO DO SO.

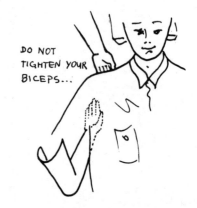

DO NOT TIGHTEN YOUR BICEPS...

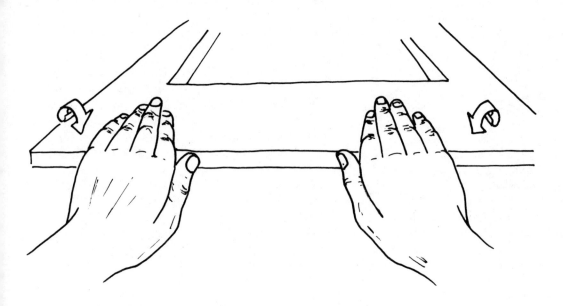

· HANDS ON THE BACK OF THE CHAIR ·

STANDING WITH A CHAIR PLACED IN FRONT OF YOU — GO INTO
MONKEY — TAKING CARE NOT TO PULL DOWN IN FRONT...
NOW — POINTING YOUR FINGERS TO THE FLOOR — BRING BOTH
HANDS UP TO REST ON THE BACK OF THE CHAIR (PALMS UP)

HAVING CHECKED YOUR
DIRECTIONS...
ROTATE YOUR THUMBS
AROUND YOUR LITTLE
FINGERS, AND BRING
THE PADS OF YOUR
FINGERS TO REST ON
THE RAIL OF THE
CHAIR...

NOW YOU ARE READY TO BRING
BOTH THUMBS AROUND AND DOWN
SO THAT THEY ARE OPPOSITE THE
INDEX FINGERS — (AS THOUGH YOU
WOULD PINCH THE CHAIR) ---

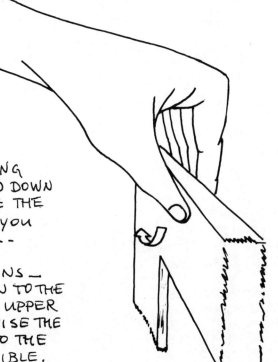

GO THROUGH YOUR DIRECTIONS —
WITH PARTICULAR ATTENTION TO THE
DIRECTION — "WIDTH ACROSS THE UPPER
ARMS AND CHEST" OTHERWISE THE
NEXT DIRECTION — "PULL TO THE
ELBOWS" — WILL NOT BE POSSIBLE.

·KNEES FORWARD AND AWAY.

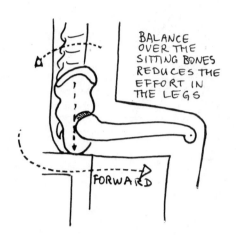

BALANCE
OVER THE
SITTING BONES
REDUCES THE
EFFORT IN
THE LEGS

FORWARD

IN FINDING BALANCE AND THEN
ALLOWING OUR WEIGHT TO
ESTABLISH THE SITTING BONES
IN THE CHAIR — WE ARE LOOKING
TO BRING THE PELVIS INTO SUCH
A POSITION THAT WE NO LONGER
NEED TO GRIP IN THE LEGS (IN
AN ATTEMPT TO HOLD OURSELVES
UP),
THE RESULT BEING THAT THIGH
CONTRACTION IS REDUCED — AND
THE LEG MUSCLES FREE INTO
THEIR NATURAL LENGTH — ALLOWING
THE KNEES, EFFECTIVELY TO GO
FORWARD---

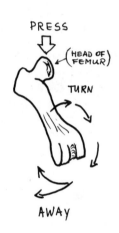

PRESS

(HEAD OF)
FEMUR)

TURN

AWAY

NOW — WHEN WE ROCK GENTLY FORWARD ON
OUR SITTING BONES (WITH THE SPINE AS ONE
PIECE) — THE ACETABULUM (OR SOCKET IN
THE PELVIS FOR THE THIGH BONE) MOVES
THE HEAD OF THE FEMUR DOWNWARDS —
CAUSING THE SHAFT OF THE BONE TO
ROTATE INWARDS, OPENING THE LEGS (AND KNEES)
AWAY FROM EACH OTHER...

THE DIRECTION OF THE BACK SPIRAL COMES
AROUND THE SIDE (GLUTEUS — VASTUS ETC)
AND ALSO HELPS TO MOVE THE KNEES OUT
PROVIDING WE KEEP THAT IN MIND AS WE
MOVE...
A USEFUL THOUGHT FOR GOING INTO AND
OUT OF MONKEY FOR EXAMPLE.

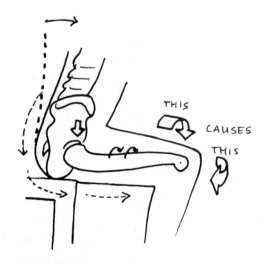

THIS

CAUSES

THIS

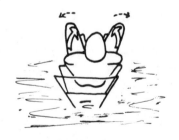

ONCE IN BALANCE — THE BACK
SPIRAL CAN BE DIRECTED
AROUND THE LEG

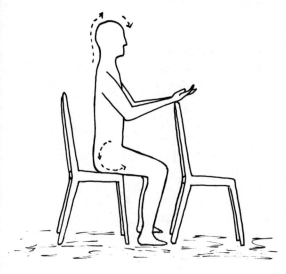

•KNEES FORWARD AND AWAY
(CONTINUED)

SITTING WITH A CHAIR PLACED
IN FRONT OF YOU...
BALANCING OVER YOUR SITTING
BONES AND ALLOWING THEM TO
TAKE YOUR WEIGHT— ASK FOR
YOUR NECK TO BE FREE SO
THAT THE HEAD CAN GO (ROLL)
FORWARD AND UP...

BRING BOTH HANDS UP TO REST
(PALMS UP) ON THE BACK OF
THE CHAIR...

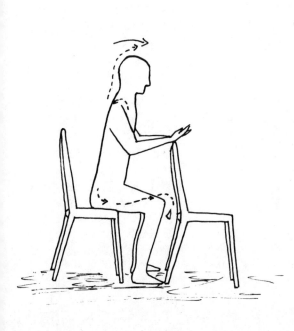

NOW— THINKING OF YOUR BACK
BEING ALL ONE PIECE, FROM
YOUR SITTING BONES UP TO
THE TOP OF YOUR HEAD (BUT
NOT HOLDING IT THAT WAY)—
COME SLIGHTLY FORWARD ON
TO YOUR HANDS AND TAKE
THE WEIGHT (NOT ON THE LEGS)

IF YOU COME TOO FAR FORWARD
YOU MAY NOT BE ABLE TO KEEP
THE LEGS FREE— WITH THE
RESULT THAT YOUR KNEES WILL
NOT GO FORWARD AND AWAY...
INSTEAD, YOU WILL GRIP AND
PULL THE THIGHS INTO THE PELVIS...

IF YOU ARE HAPPY WITH THE
FREEDOM IN THE LEGS WHILE
USING YOUR HANDS INSTEAD...
PULL TO THE ELBOWS (THINK OF
THE SPINE ADVANCING BETWEEN
YOUR SHOULDERS).

• USING THE WHISPERED AH — TO HELP YOU MOVE WITHOUT PULLING DOWN.

A VERY IMPORTANT PART OF DOING A WHISPERED AH IS TO USE THE OPPORTUNITY TO OBSERVE WHETHER YOU ARE INCLINED TO PULL YOUR HEAD BACK AND/OR TO PULL DOWN IN FRONT AS YOU EXHALE — SAYING "AH" IS A GOOD MEANS WHEREBY YOU CAN OBSERVE ANY KIND OF CHANGES IN THE SOUND (OR THE MECHANISM FOR THE CREATION OF THAT SOUND) WHEN YOU VOCALISE.

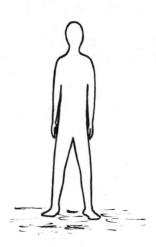

AND SO — WITH THIS IN MIND, BEGIN BY STANDING WITH YOUR FEET A LITTLE WIDER APART THAN NORMAL — BUT NOT SO WIDE THAT YOUR DIRECTIONS ARE DIFFICULT TO MANAGE...

THEN — DIRECTING AS MUCH AS YOU CAN FROM ONE HEEL (LET US SAY.. THE RIGHT FOOT) — FLICK THE OTHER FOOT (LEFT) IN TO THE SIDE SO THAT YOUR FEET ARE NOW CLOSER TOGETHER (IDEALLY UNDER BOTH HIP JOINTS)

NOW — START AGAIN WITH YOUR FEET A LITTLE WIDER APART THAN USUAL.....

AND — AS YOU DIRECT UP FROM ONE HEEL — CHOOSE AN OUT-BREATH (ANY OUT-BREATH) AND WHISPER AH...WHILE AT THE SAME TIME FLICKING THE OTHER FOOT IN TO THE SIDE...

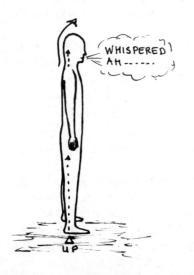

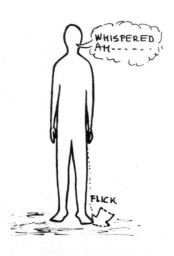

YOU ARE LOOKING FOR AN EXTRA LITTLE BIT OF "UP" FROM THE AH...
YET AT THE SAME TIME YOU WILL NOTICE HOW VERY EASY IT IS TO PULL DOWN...

NOW REPEAT THE WHOLE THING ON THE OTHER SIDE.

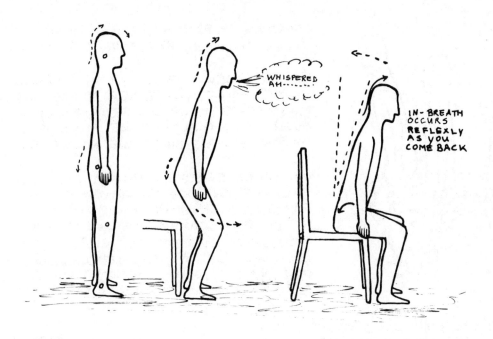

WHISPERED AH.....

IN-BREATH OCCURS REFLEXLY AS YOU COME BACK

• THE WHISPERED AH — AND GOING FROM STANDING INTO SITTING.

A REASONABLE UNDERSTANDING AND EXPERIENCE OF THE WHISPERED AH IN ITS OWN RIGHT WILL PROVE VALUABLE IN THESE ACTIVITIES.

WE BEGIN BY STANDING IN FRONT OF A CHAIR AND LOOKING FOR FREEDOM THROUGHOUT — (NOT ONLY THE NECK, BUT ALSO THE PELVIS — HIPS — KNEES — ANKLES ETC..) --- SO TAKE YOUR TIME TO ESTABLISH THIS FREEDOM.

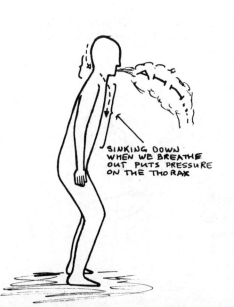

SINKING DOWN WHEN WE BREATHE OUT PUTS PRESSURE ON THE THORAX

AS WE PREPARE TO SIT — THE THOUGHT IS NATURALLY GOING TO BE A "DOWN" THOUGHT --- SO USE A WHISPERED AH TO PICK UP ON ANY PULLING DOWN AS YOU ALLOW YOUR KNEES TO GO FORWARD AND AWAY---

THEN — AS YOU COME INTO THE CHAIR AND BRING YOUR WEIGHT OVER THE SITTING BONES — ALLOW THE IN-BREATH TO TAKE PLACE AS NATURALLY AND REFLEXLY AS POSSIBLE.

NOW USE THE WHISPERED AH TO TAKE YOU OUT OF THE CHAIR.

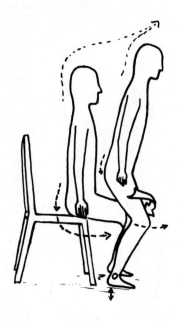

'STANDING UP FROM A CHAIR — USING
KNEES FORWARD AND AWAY.

THE NET RESULT OF BEING IN BALANCE
IS THAT WE NO LONGER NEED TO USE OUR
MUSCLES TO HOLD US FROM FALLING
OVER, AND THE MORE WE FREE INTO
BALANCE.. THE MORE WE RELEASE...

SO — WHILE SEATED — MAINTAIN YOUR
BALANCE BY ROCKING YOUR SKULL
FORWARD OVER YOUR A/O JOINT...
AT THIS POINT — TAKE CARE NOT TO PUSH
YOURSELF OUT OF THE CHAIR WITH
YOUR LEGS (OR BACK). INSTEAD — ALLOW THE
FORWARD (AND UP) MOMENTUM TO
SCOOP YOU OUT AND ON TO YOUR HEELS.

OUR LEG MUSCLES DO NOT
GO IN A STRAIGHT LINE
FROM ONE END TO THE OTHER.
INSTEAD — THEY "SPIRAL"...
AROUND FROM THE BACK
DOWN THE SIDE AND
OVER THE FRONT OF
THE LEG TO THE INSIDE.
(AT THE KNEE)...
SO WHEN WE ALLOW OUR
WEIGHT TO GO INTO THE
CHAIR THROUGH THE
SITTING BONES, WE ARE

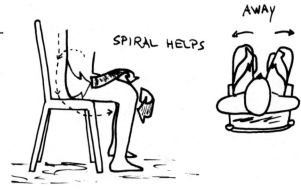

SPIRAL HELPS

AWAY

FEEDING INTO THE BACK SPIRAL   AND ALLOWING THE KNEES
TO GO FORWARD AND AWAY (EVEN DURING STANDING).

THERE MAY BE A POINT WHERE YOU WILL NEED TO TRUST THAT
ONCE YOUR WEIGHT SHIFTS (IN BALANCE) FROM THE SITTING
BONES — FORWARD ON
TO YOUR HEELS —
THE BALANCE WILL
STILL BE INTACT,
AND STANDING WILL BE
ALMOST EFFORTLESS.

OTHERWISE — YOU WILL
PULL YOUR LEGS INTO
THE PELVIS — DISTURB
THE BALANCE — AND
SET OFF A REACTION
IN COMPENSATION
FROM HEAD TO FOOT.

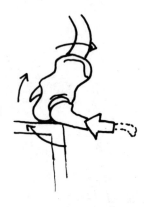

FORWARD AS
YOU STAND

• SHOULDERS BACK AND DOWN – AND HANDS ON THE BACK OF THE CHAIR.

WHILE SEATED – BEGIN BY CHECKING OVER YOUR DIRECTIONS.
NECK FREE – HEAD FORWARD AND UP AND YOUR WEIGHT OVER THE SITTING BONES ...
NOW BRING BOTH HANDS UP TO REST (PALMS UP) ON THE BACK OF A CHAIR PLACED IN FRONT OF YOU...
THEN – AFTER GOING OVER YOUR DIRECTIONS ONCE MORE – COME SLIGHTLY FORWARD (ROCKING ON THE SITTING BONES) TAKING THE WEIGHT ON YOUR HANDS...
YOUR LEGS WILL BE FREE ENOUGH (NOT TAKING WEIGHT) TO ALLOW YOUR KNEES TO GO FORWARD AND AWAY...
NOW ASK FOR WIDTH ACROSS THE UPPER ARMS – RELEASING THE SHOULDERS BACK AND DOWN (INTO YOUR BACK)...
WITHOUT THESE CONDITIONS, "PULLING TO THE ELBOWS" IS NOT GOING TO BE POSSIBLE.

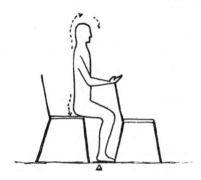 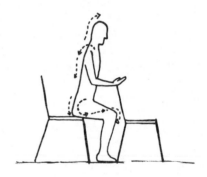

BEFORE WIDENING TAKES PLACE – WE MUST ACHIEVE RELEASE AND LENGTH IN THE PECTORALS, FREEING THEM FROM PULLING THE SHOULDERS FORWARD AND INTO THE CHEST.

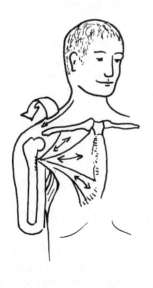 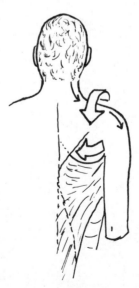

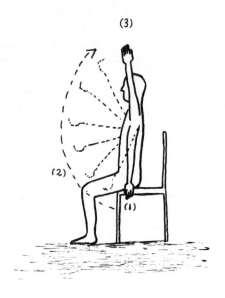

· MOVING THE ARMS IN A CIRCLE ·

SITTING ON A CHAIR _ AND BALANCING ON BOTH SITTING BONES WITH YOUR HANDS DOWN BY YOUR SIDE...

POINT YOUR FINGERS TO THE FLOOR (ALMOST AS IF YOU COULD TOUCH THE GROUND) _ ASK FOR LENGTH FROM YOUR EARS TO YOUR FINGER-TIPS...

CONTINUING TO POINT_BRING YOUR HAND OUT TO IN FRONT OF YOU_ (NOTICE HOW YOUR BALANCE CHANGES. AS MORE WEIGHT COMES FORWARD, YOU COME BACK ON YOUR SITTING BONES)...

FOLLOW ON TO ABOVE YOUR HEAD_ BUT NOT SO HIGH THAT YOU END UP STICKING YOUR NECK AND HEAD OUT _ GO ONLY AS FAR AS YOUR ABILITY TO RELEASE WILL ALLOW...

NOW BRING YOUR HAND OUT TO THE SIDE _ POINTING STILL _ (NOTICE HOW THE SHIFT OF WEIGHT MAY TEMPT YOU TO BEND THE SPINE TO THE OTHER SIDE _ INSTEAD OF BALANCING YOUR HEAD AND THE REST OF YOUR BODY SLIGHTLY OVER THE OPPOSITE SITTING BONE)

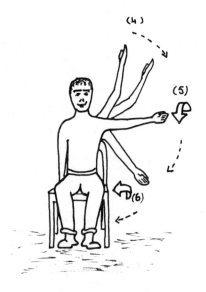

ONCE OUT TO THE SIDE _ ROTATE YOUR THUMB AROUND YOUR LITTLE FINGER TO FACE THE PALM OF YOUR HAND FORWARD...

THEN_AS YOU CONTINUE DOWN TO THE SIDE_ALLOW THE HAND TO TURN_TO A POINT OF REST DOWN BY THE SIDE ...

NOW REPEAT EACH STEP ON THE OTHER SIDE...

REMEMBER _ MOVE BY WAY OF RELEASE RATHER THAN EFFORT.

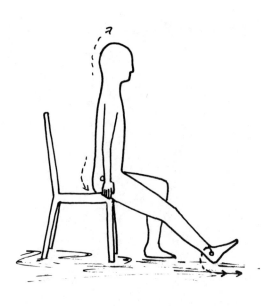

• DIRECTING YOUR HEELS AWAY FROM YOUR SITTING BONES.

SITTING ON THE EDGE OF THE CHAIR (WITH ENOUGH SPACE TO SUPPORT THE SITTING BONES) — IMAGINE YOU COULD POINT WITH YOUR HEEL...

THEN — DIRECTING FROM AS BALANCED A POSITION AS IS AVAILABLE TO YOU — SEND YOUR HEEL ALONG THE FLOOR AWAY FROM YOUR SITTING BONE...

NOW — WITH YOUR LEG STRAIGHT OUT IN FRONT OF YOU — ASK FOR AS MUCH LENGTH AS POSSIBLE BETWEEN THE HEEL AND THE SITTING BONE (TAKING THE PRECAUTION NOT TO TRY TO PUSH)...

SLOWLY BRING YOUR HEEL BACK TO UNDER THE KNEE WHILE KEEPING AS MUCH LENGTH AS POSSIBLE IN THE PROCESS...

NOW REPEAT THE PROCEDURE WITH YOUR OTHER LEG...

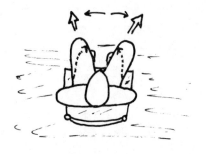

THEN — ONCE YOU HAVE BROUGHT YOUR OTHER LEG BACK TO UNDER THE KNEE — MOVE BOTH KNEES APART FROM EACH OTHER OPENING AND THEN CLOSING YOUR LEGS — WHILE BALANCING ON YOUR SITTING BONES.

YOU COULD REPEAT THE GAME AGAIN IF YOU WISH. THEN — ONCE IT IS COMPLETED COME INTO STANDING, SENDING YOUR KNEES FORWARD AND AWAY.

THIS CAN BE USEFUL FOR VOICE USERS (ACTORS, SINGERS AND SO ON) BECAUSE ONE OF THE THINGS THEY TEND TO DO, IS TO USE THEIR LEGS AS THOUGH THEY COULD SQUEEZE THE SOUND OUT — DEPRESSING THE LARYNX.

RELEASING THE BACK - BY TAKING
YOUR WEIGHT ON TO YOUR HANDS.

THIS WAS A PROCEDURE F. M.
USED WITH HIS PUPILS TO GET
THE BACK WORKING.

SITTING IN THE CHAIR WITH YOUR
HANDS RESTING (PALMS UP) ON
YOUR LEGS...

GO THROUGH YOUR DIRECTIONS,
LENGTHENING AND WIDENING
AS YOU BALANCE OVER YOUR
SITTING BONES, FREEING THE
LEGS AS YOUR SEAT TAKES
THE WEIGHT...

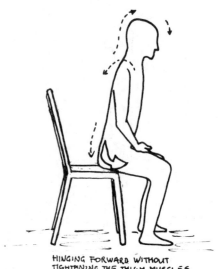

HINGING FORWARD WITHOUT
TIGHTENING THE THIGH MUSCLES

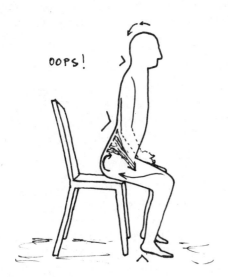

OOPS!

NOW HINGE FORWARD WHILE
GRADUALLY TAKING THE
WEIGHT ON TO YOUR HANDS -
THROUGH INTO THE ARMS AND
THEN INTO THE BACK...

MAKE SURE THAT YOUR
BOTTOM IS STILL RESTING ON
THE CHAIR, AND NOT LIFTING
OFF. (BY PULLING THE PELVIS
AND LUMBAR SPINE FORWARD
WITH THE LEG MUSCLES)...
TAKE IT SLOWLY, OBSERVING
AS YOU GO...

IF YOU MANAGE TO KEEP THE LEGS
FREE, YOU WILL BE ABLE TO MOVE
WITHOUT   ING THE DYNAMIC
IN THE BACK MUSCLES...

ALL GOING WELL - ONCE FORWARD,
GIVE SOME THOUGHT TO THE IDEA
OF ADVANCING YOUR SPINE
BETWEEN THE SHOULDERS -
AND CONNECT YOUR ARMS INTO
THE BACK...

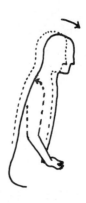

THE EXTENSORS OF THE BACK CAN NOW BE USED AS YOU STAND UP.

• USING YOUR BACK — WHILE TAKING THE RAIL OF A CHAIR IN YOUR HANDS.

FOLLOWING PREVIOUS INSTRUCTIONS BRING BOTH HANDS UP AND ON TO THE BACK OF THE CHAIR PLACED IN FRONT OF YOU ...

TAKING THE RAIL BETWEEN YOUR THUMB AND INDEX FINGER (ALONG WITH THE OTHER FINGERS) IN CORTICAL OPPOSITION ...

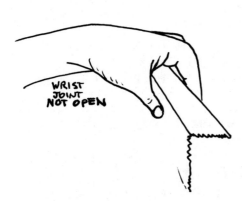

WRIST JOINT NOT OPEN

SEND YOUR THUMB TOWARDS THE FLOOR — FREEING THE WRIST AND BRINGING IT AROUND AND DOWN (WITH THE THUMB) ...

GRADUALLY ROCK FORWARD ON THE SITTING BONES — AND USE YOUR HANDS TO TAKE THE WEIGHT THROUGH AND INTO YOUR BACK

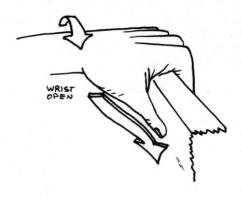

WRIST OPEN

ASK FOR LENGTH IN THE EXTENSORS FROM YOUR HANDS TO YOUR ELBOWS — UP THE BACK OF THE ARMS AND INTO YOUR SHOULDER BLADES (THINKING OF FLATTENING THEM INTO YOUR BACK)
MUSCULAR EFFORT RESULTS IN THORACIC RIGIDITY — SO DO NOT REMAIN IN THIS POSITION FOR TOO LONG ...

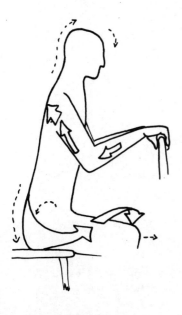

THIS IS NOT THE SAME AS "THORACIC EXPANSION" — WHICH WAS USED AS AN EXERCISE DURING VOICE TRAINING .. THE PERSON WOULD PULL ON THE CHAIR — AND FEEL AS THOUGH THE CHEST WAS EXPANDING ... NOT UNLIKE WHAT HAPPENS WHEN WE SIMPLY PULL OUR SHOULDERS BACK.

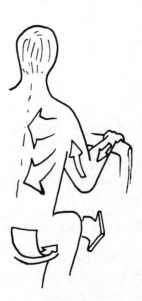

• USING YOUR BACK — IN MONKEY — WITH YOUR HANDS ON THE TEACHING TABLE.

WHEN GOING INTO MONKEY, WE ALL HAVE A TENDENCY TO SHORTEN RATHER THAN LENGTHEN IN STATURE.
SO — WITH THIS IN MIND — GO INTO MONKEY (AT THE EDGE OF YOUR TEACHING TABLE)...

NOW — POINTING YOUR FINGERS — BRING YOUR HANDS UP TO REST (PALMS DOWN)...

OUT OF INTEREST — ASK YOURSELF IS THE WEIGHT EVENLY DISTRIBUTED? — OR ARE YOU TOO FAR FORWARD (OR BACK)? OR MAYBE MORE ON ONE SIDE THAN THE OTHER? —
BEING OUT OF BALANCE REQUIRES EXTRA EFFORT TO KEEP US FROM FALLING OVER — WE WILL END UP HOLDING ON IN THE LEGS AND SHORTENING THE ANKLE, KNEE AND HIP JOINT SPACES, AND ALSO THE INTERVERTEBRAL (DIS) JOINTS...

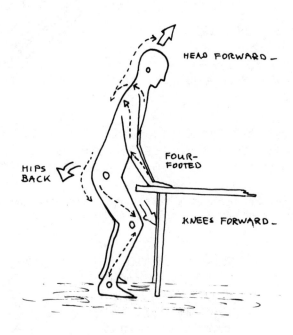

HEAD FORWARD —

FOUR-FOOTED

HIPS BACK

KNEES FORWARD —

SO — ALLOW THE PALMS OF YOUR HANDS TO REST ON THE TABLE — AND USE THE HEELS OF YOUR HANDS TO LENGTHEN AWAY FROM GRAVITY (IN THE SAME WAY YOU WOULD USE THE HEELS OF YOUR FEET)---

NOW ALLOW YOUR KNEES TO GO FORWARD — TAKING THE WEIGHT THROUGH THE HANDS AND ARMS INTO YOUR BACK...

YOU ARE LOOKING FOR AN ELASTIC CONNECTION BETWEEN YOUR TOES AND YOUR HEAD — AS YOU COME INTO STANDING.

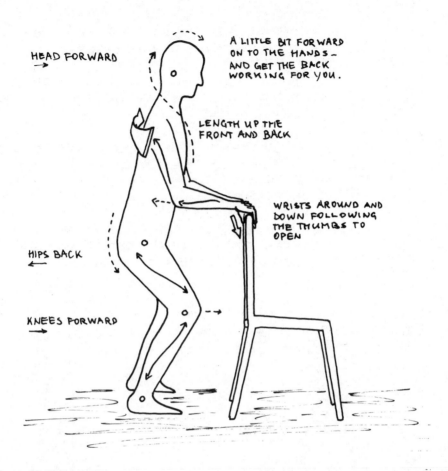

HEAD FORWARD

A LITTLE BIT FORWARD
ON TO THE HANDS—
AND GET THE BACK
WORKING FOR YOU.

LENGTH UP THE
FRONT AND BACK

WRISTS AROUND AND
DOWN FOLLOWING
THE THUMBS TO
OPEN

HIPS BACK

KNEES FORWARD

• USING YOUR BACK — IN MONKEY — WITH YOUR HANDS ON THE BACK
OF A CHAIR.

STANDING IN FRONT OF A CHAIR AND DIRECTING YOURSELF
INTO BALANCE—SEND YOUR HEAD AND KNEES FORWARD, AND
YOUR HIPS BACK, TO GO INTO MONKEY...
(MONKEY IS NOT A FIXED POSITION. RATHER, IT IS FLEXIBLE
AND OPEN TO CHANGE)...

NOW— BRING YOUR HANDS UP TO THE BACK OF THE CHAIR...

THEN—TAKE THE RAIL BETWEEN YOUR THUMB AND FINGERS—
FREEING YOUR WRISTS BY SENDING THE THUMBS DOWN TO
THE FLOOR...

AT THIS STAGE—WE ARE LOOKING FOR LENGTH FROM THE
HIPS TO THE KNEES — FROM THE ANKLES TO THE KNEES —
LENGTH UP THE FRONT — LENGTH UP THE BACK — WIDTH
ACROSS THE UPPER ARMS (FRONT AND BACK) — PULLING TO
THE ELBOWS — NECK FREE AND SO ON——
AS IF YOU WERE FOUR-FOOTED (YOUR ARMS FEEDING INTO THE BACK)
GENTLY BRING YOUR WEIGHT ON TO THE HANDS BY SENDING
YOUR KNEES A LITTLE MORE FORWARD —DIRECT— THEN STAND.

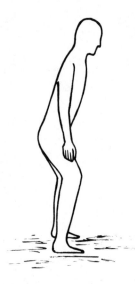

• LIFTING A CHAIR — USING YOUR BACK, AND NOT TIGHTENING YOUR BICEPS.

BEING CONSCIOUS THAT YOU ARE GOING TO LIFT A CHAIR CAN BE ENOUGH TO PULL YOU DOWN —

SO — KEEPING THIS IN MIND — LOOK AT THE CHAIR'S CENTRE OF BALANCE — AND, DIRECTING AWAY FROM THAT POINT — GO INTO MONKEY...

NOW SEND YOUR HEAD FORWARD — AND YOUR HIPS BACK EVEN MORE — BRINGING YOURSELF INTO A DEEPER MONKEY...

RESTING YOUR HANDS ON OR NEAR THE CENTRE OF BALANCE — PAUSE AND CHECK YOUR DIRECTIONS...

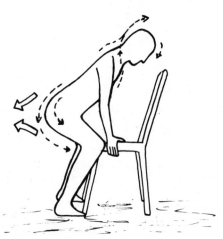

ANKLES AND HIPS FREE SO THAT YOUR KNEES CAN GO FORWARD — FEEDING YOUR ARMS INTO YOUR BACK (AS BEFORE) — SAY "NO" TO LIFTING, INSTEAD, SIMPLY COME INTO STANDING — TAKING THE CHAIR WITH YOU... OBSERVING ANY PULLING IN YOUR BICEPS DURING THE MOVEMENT.

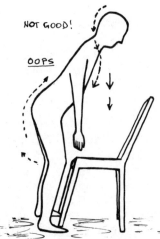

NOT GOOD!

OOPS

TAKE YOUR TIME WITH THIS GAME — BECAUSE IF YOU JUST GO AHEAD AND DO IT, YOU ARE SURE TO PULL YOURSELF OUT OF BALANCE — COMING OVER ON TO YOUR TOES AND STIFFENING IN THE JOINTS.

• STEPPING UP — GOING UP STAIRS — OR FOOTPATH — ETC.

THROUGHOUT THESE ACTIVITIES IT IS USEFUL TO KEEP IN MIND THE FACT THAT WE ALL TEND TO LEAN FORWARD WHEN LIFTING A LEG — AND IN SO DOING, PULL DOWN IN FRONT...

SO— WE BEGIN WITH OUR FEET A LITTLE CLOSER TOGETHER THAN NORMAL — AND, AS FAR AS WE CAN TELL, ALLOWING OUR WEIGHT TO GO THROUGH THE FLOOR VIA THE HEELS AND THE OUTSIDE EDGES OF THE FEET ...

NOW — USING THE BACK SPIRAL — SEND YOUR KNEE FORWARD (BENDING IT), LIFTING YOUR HEEL OFF THE FLOOR AND ALSO BENDING THE FOOT AT YOUR TOES...

BEING CAREFUL NOT TO PUSH YOURSELF OFF BALANCE FLICK THAT FOOT FORWARD (FROM THE BEND IN THE FOOT)...

FINALLY BRING THE FOOT BACK TO THE SIDE BY USING THE BALL OF THE FOOT (TO PUSH OFF FROM) — NOW REPEAT ON OTHER SIDE.

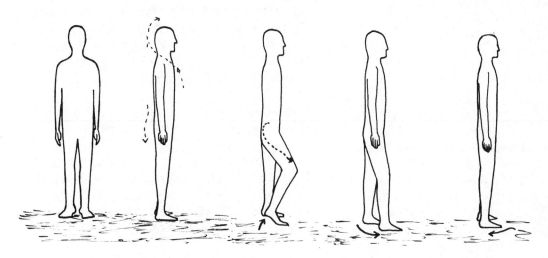

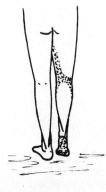

THIS TIME — PLACE A TELEPHONE BOOK (OR A STEP) IN FRONT OF YOUR TOES (ALMOST TOUCHING)

NOW — FOLLOW THE INSTRUCTIONS ABOVE — BUT INSTEAD OF FLICKING YOUR FOOT FORWARD. FLICK IT UP AND ON TO THE STEP IN FRONT OF YOU...

WITHOUT PAUSING — BRING YOUR FOOT BACK TO THE SIDE — AND REPEAT ON THE OTHER SIDE.

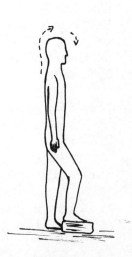

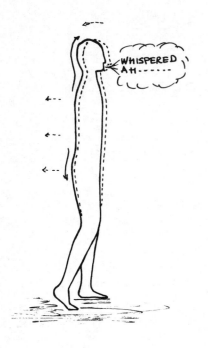

· USING THE WHISPERED AH TO MOVE YOU BACKWARDS.

THE FIRST THING WE NEED BEFORE ATTEMPTING A WHISPERED AH — IS FREEDOM IN THE ANKLES — KNEES AND HIPS ETC.. AND BALANCED ON TOP OF ALL OF THAT --- THE HEAD GOING FORWARD AND UP OVER A FREE ATLANTO-OCCIPITAL JOINT.
NOW — ONCE YOU HAVE CHECKED OVER YOUR DIRECTIONS, AND YOU ARE SATISFIED THAT YOU ARE WELL ESTABLISHED ON THE GROUND — PICK AN OUT-BREATH — (SMILING IN THE EYES — THE TIP OF THE TONGUE TO THE TOP OF THE LOWER TEETH — DROPPING THE JAW AND WIDENING THE GAP BETWEEN YOUR BACK TEETH) — DO A WHISPERED AH — AND ALLOW IT TO PUSH YOU BACK ON YOUR HEELS (LIKE THE LID OF A BOX) — UNTIL IT IS INEVITABLE THAT YOU TAKE A STEP BACKWARDS ---

EVENTUALLY ALLOWING IT TO BECOME A WALK — DO A SERIES OF "AHS"...

IT IS VERY EASY TO TIGHTEN UNDER THE CHIN AND PULL DOWN — WHILE WALKING BACKWARDS — SO USING THE WHISPERED AH TO MONITOR — AND HELP ELIMINATE IT.

AS AN ALTERNATIVE TO AN AH ... DO AN "UM". ONCE YOUR BALANCE HAS TAKEN THE PRESSURE OFF THE RIBS ... IT IS THE SAME AS THE "AH" — BUT WITH YOUR LIPS CLOSED.

NOW SEATED — USING THE SITTING BONES IN THE SAME WAY AS WE USE OUR HEELS (FOR BALANCE AND SUPPORT)

ANKLES, KNEES AND HIPS FREE — (RELEASE UNDER THE CHIN) ... PICK AN OUT-BREATH AND DO AN AH... ALLOWING IT TO SEND YOU BACK A LITTLE MORE ON YOUR SITTING BONES WHILE COMING UP IN FRONT.

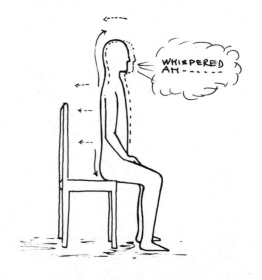

PART THREE

TERM ONE
FIRST HALF

BENDING ONE KNEE AFTER THE OTHER — AND LIFTING A FOOT OFF THE GROUND.

①. STANDING WITH YOUR FEET CLOSER TOGETHER THAN HIP-WIDTH AND YOUR EYES LIVELY...
BRING YOUR WEIGHT SLIGHTLY MORE OVER ONE HEEL THAN THE OTHER — TAKING CARE NOT TO SHIFT YOUR PELVIS TO THAT SIDE...
NOW — ON THE OTHER SIDE — THINK OF LENGTHENING FROM YOUR HIP TO YOUR KNEE — SENDING THAT KNEE FORWARD — BENDING AT THE BALL OF YOUR FOOT AND BRINGING YOUR HEEL OFF THE GROUND IN THE PROCESS — AND THEN SEND YOUR HEEL TO THE FLOOR, AND BACK TO WHERE YOU STARTED...

②. REPEAT THE INSTRUCTIONS ON THE OTHER SIDE.

③. GO THROUGH THE SAME PROCEDURES, ONLY THIS TIME — GOING FROM ONE SIDE TO THE OTHER WITHOUT STOPPING

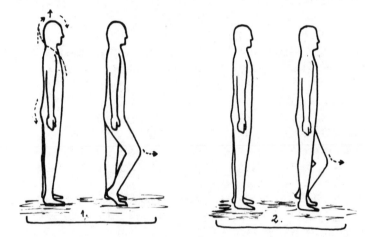 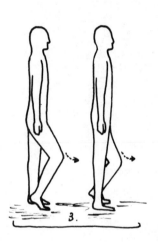

THIS TIME — GO AS FAR AS SENDING YOUR KNEE FORWARD, AND ONCE YOUR FOOT IS BENT...
LIFT IT OF THE GROUND.
N.B. YOU MUST BE DIRECTING VERY CLEARLY FROM THE OTHER HEEL — OTHERWISE YOU WILL PUSH THE PELVIS OUT TO THE SIDE — USE YOUR SHOULDERS — AND/OR — WOBBLE ABOUT.

TAKE THE IDEA INTO WALKING — THINKING OF SENDING YOUR KNEES FORWARD FROM HIPS — THROUGH THIGHS — TO KNEES (INSTEAD OF BALL OF FOOT TO KNEE)

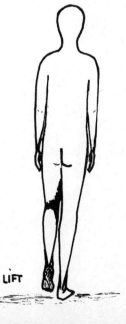

LIFT

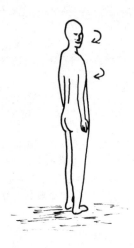

• USING YOUR EYES TO TURN YOUR HEAD —
AND THEN TO TURN YOUR BODY

WHILE STANDING — LOOK TOWARDS THE RIGHT
SHOULDER (WITHOUT TURNING YOUR HEAD)...
THEN ALLOW THE HEAD TO FOLLOW...
CONTINUE BY TURNING THE BODY AS IF TO
LOOK BEHIND YOU (CAREFUL NOT TO PULL)...
NOW COME BACK TO LOOKING IN FRONT OF
YOU AND REPEAT ON YOUR LEFT SIDE —

NOTICE HOW YOU WILL BE LOOKING AT THE
SHOULDER WITH THE SAME SIDE EYE —
THE OTHER EYE WILL ONLY SEE YOUR NOSE.

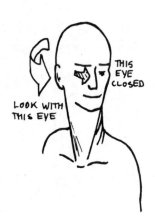

LOOK WITH
THIS EYE

THIS
EYE
CLOSED

THIS TIME — CLOSE YOUR LEFT EYE..., AND USE
YOUR RIGHT EYE TO "PUSH" YOUR NOSE —
AND THEN YOUR HEAD AROUND — SO THAT
EVENTUALLY YOU ARE TURNED TO YOUR
LEFT AS IF TO LOOK BEHIND YOU...
NOW COME BACK TO LOOKING IN FRONT OF
YOU, AND — CLOSING YOUR RIGHT EYE —
REPEAT BY USING YOUR LEFT EYE TO TURN
TO THE RIGHT...

NOW STANDING WITH YOUR FEET CLOSE
TOGETHER — POINT YOUR FINGERS TO THE
FLOOR — THEN TURN YOUR HANDS INTO THE
ANATOMICAL POSITION...
BRING THEM OUT TO THE SIDE (SLOWLY)
UNTIL THEY ARE JUST ABOVE SHOULDER
LEVEL, AND YOUR PALMS FACING UPWARD...
NOW LOOK TO YOUR RIGHT AS BEFORE —
ALLOWING THE BODY TO FOLLOW — THEN
BACK TO IN FRONT OF YOU, AND THEN THE
OTHER SIDE...

THIS TIME — WHILE SEATED — FOLLOW
THE INSTRUCTIONS ABOVE.

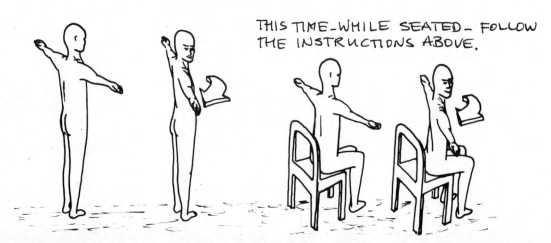

• SITTING AND STANDING - WHILE USING YOUR HANDS TO HELP DIRECT YOUR PELVIS BACK AND DOWN.

PLACE YOUR HANDS ON EITHER SIDE OF THE PELVIS (ILIAC CREST) WITH YOUR FINGERS POINTING DOWN AND BACK...
WE ARE LOOKING TO DISCOURAGE ANY TILTING FORWARD OF THE PELVIS AS WE MOVE IN AND OUT OF THE CHAIR...

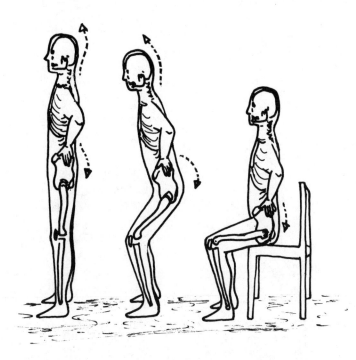

STANDING IN FRONT OF A CHAIR...
ALLOW YOUR HEELS TO TAKE YOUR WEIGHT, WHILE SENDING YOUR HEAD FORWARD AND UP - AND YOUR PELVIS BACK AND DOWN...
NOW SEND YOUR HEAD FORWARD KNEES FORWARD AND HIPS BACK TO GO INTO THE CHAIR... USE YOUR HANDS TO OBSERVE.

"HIPS BACK AND DOWN" IS NOT SO MUCH THE.. HIP JOINTS BACK - BUT THE PELVIS ITSELF...
OTHERWISE YOU COULD ACTUALLY TILT THE PELVIS FORWARD - - -

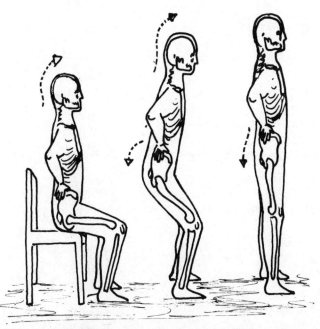

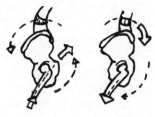

HIP JOINTS BACK......   PELVIS BACK....

NOW YOU ARE SEATED... COME INTO STANDING, OBSERVING AS YOU GO.

· HANDS BEHIND YOUR BACK – AND GOING INTO–
AND OUT OF THE CHAIR.

WHILE STANDING – POINT YOUR FINGERS TO
THE FLOOR ...
GRADUALLY BRING ONE HAND AT A TIME – TO
BEHIND YOUR BACK (AS YOU BEND AT THE
ELBOWS, DIRECT THEM TOWARDS THE FLOOR
TO AVOID LIFTING THE SHOULDERS)...

IT IS NOT NECESSARY TO HOLD YOUR ELBOWS
IN YOUR HANDS – DO NOT FORCE IT – GO ONLY
AS FAR AS IS COMFORTABLE ...

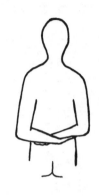

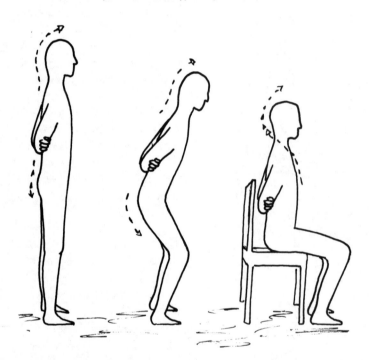

NOW THAT YOU ARE
SET UP – MAKE
FULL USE OF THE
EXTRA WEIGHT TO
THE BACK BY
ALLOWING IT TO BE
TAKEN BY THE
HEELS ...
THEN – SENDING
YOUR HEAD
FORWARD AND UP–
TAKE YOURSELF
INTO THE CHAIR...

OBSERVE AS YOU
MOVE ...

NOW THAT YOU ARE IN THE CHAIR – ALLOW
THE EXTRA WEIGHT AT THE BACK TO GO
THROUGH THE SITTING BONES (AS IF
YOU COULD DROP YOUR BOTTOM INTO
THE CHAIR) – LOOK FOR LENGTH UP THE
FRONT BY SENDING YOUR HEAD
FORWARD AND UP ...
ROCK GENTLY BACK AND THEN COME INTO
STANDING.

WITH YOUR ARMS BEHIND YOUR BACK –
BE CAREFUL YOU DONT STICK YOUR
CHIN OUT BY PULLING YOUR HEAD
BACK – OR STICK YOUR BOTTOM OUT,
ETC ... ETC ... ETC ...

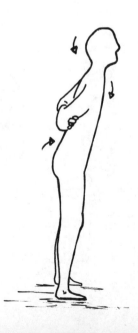

· LIFTING A CHAIR – AND LIFTING A LEG.

GO INTO MONKEY IN FRONT OF A CHAIR ...
THEN – WITHOUT THINKING YOU ARE GOING TO LIFT IT – GO INTO
A DEEPER MONKEY PLACING YOUR HANDS ON THE EDGES ...
NOW – TAKE THE CHAIR'S WEIGHT INTO YOUR HEELS VIA THE
EXTENSOR SURFACE OF YOUR ARMS, BACK, BUTTOCKS AND THE
BACKS OF YOUR THIGHS AND LEGS – STAND.

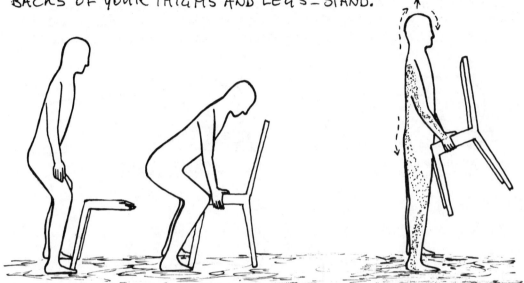

LIFTING A PUPIL'S LEG IS THE SAME, IN THAT WE DO NOT WANT TO
TIGHTEN THE BICEPS, BUT TO FEED THE WEIGHT THROUGH OUR
ARMS AND BACK INTO THE HEELS (FOR STRONGER DIRECTIONS) ...
SO – WITH ONE HAND UNDER THE BACK OF THE KNEE (AS SHOWN),
AND THE OTHER UNDER THE FOOT (PROMOTING LENGTH FROM THE
HEEL WITH YOUR MIDDLE FINGER – LIFT THE LEG ...

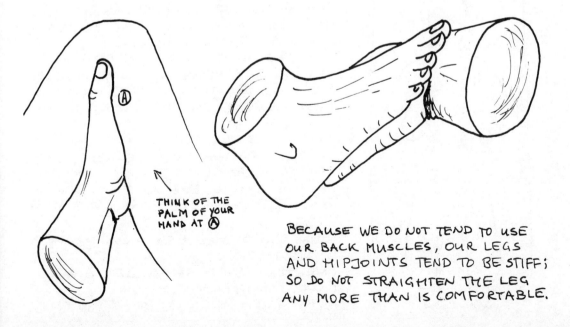

THINK OF THE
PALM OF YOUR
HAND AT Ⓐ

BECAUSE WE DO NOT TEND TO USE
OUR BACK MUSCLES, OUR LEGS
AND HIP JOINTS TEND TO BE STIFF;
SO DO NOT STRAIGHTEN THE LEG
ANY MORE THAN IS COMFORTABLE.

· SHOULDER WORK — AND BOOK HEIGHT .

THIS IS A CONTINUATION FROM LIFTING THE LEGS — SINCE THE
LUMBAR AREA OF THE SPINE TENDS TO RELEASE (TOWARDS
THE TABLE) AFTER LEG WORK...
MAKE SURE THAT THE BOOKS ARE NOT TOO LOW FOR THE PUPIL'S
HEAD, BECAUSE THE THORACIC OR KYPHOTIC CURVE WILL NOT
ALLOW THE NECK TO RELEASE AS THE LUMBAR CURVE DOES...
AND SO THE PECTORALS, L. DORSI AND NECK MUSCLES WILL
HAVE TIGHTENED — MAKING FURTHER WORK VERY DIFFICULT...

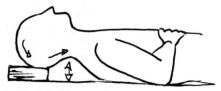

BOOKS TOO LOW —
NECK CURVE ARCHES

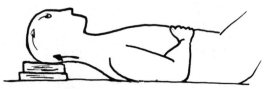

CORRECT HEIGHT —
PROMOTES EXTENSION

NOW YOU CAN
TAKE THE
SHOULDER

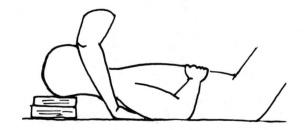

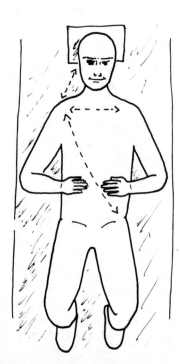

ONCE YOU ARE SATISFIED ABOUT THE
BOOK HEIGHT — PLACE ONE HAND UNDER
THE SHOULDER (COMFORTABLY) — AND
THE OTHER HAND OVER THE PECTORALS
(JUST AT THE SHOULDER)...
PROCEED WITH YOUR DIRECTIONS —
ASKING FOR RELEASE IN YOURSELF —
AND — AS A RESULT — IN YOUR PUPIL...
THEN REPEAT ON THE OTHER SIDE.

IN PREPARATION FOR THE NEXT GAME —
ASK YOUR PUPIL TO DIRECT (OR THINK
OF) THE SHOULDERS AS FAR AWAY AS
POSSIBLE FROM THE EARS (ONE AT A
TIME)...
THEN THE SHOULDERS AWAY FROM
EACHOTHER...
AND THEN EACH SHOULDER AWAY
FROM THE OPPOSITE HIP...
IF THE PUPIL "DOES" IT, DO NOT GO ON.

· STICKING THE TONGUE OUT — AND WHISPERED AH (IN THE SEMI-SUPINE POSITION).

STANDING AT THE HEAD OF YOUR PUPIL — GO INTO MONKEY AND BRING YOUR HANDS UP TO REST (PALMS DOWN ON THE TABLE) EITHER SIDE OF YOUR PUPIL'S HEAD...
HAVING GONE OVER YOUR DIRECTIONS — PLACE BOTH HANDS AT THE THE PUPIL'S HEAD AS IF TO TAKE IT...
AT THIS POINT, YOU WANT TO ENCOURAGE LENGTH IN YOUR PUPIL — SO PULL TO THE ELBOWS (SOFTEN AND LENGTHEN THE FOREARM AND THE EXTENSORS AND FLEXORS OF THE HAND), AND RELEASE AND WIDEN THE CHEST (AND UPPER ARMS)...

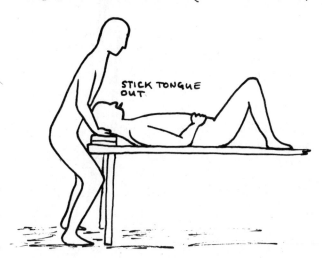

STICK TONGUE OUT

IF YOUR PUPIL'S TONGUE IS FREE, IT MAY TEND TO FALL TO THE BACK OF THE THROAT — SO ASK THE PUPIL TO MOVE IT AROUND THE TEETH... THEN — IF THE NECK IS STILL FREE AND THE HEAD NOT PULLED BACK — ASK YOUR PUPIL TO STICK HIS OR HER TONGUE OUT — WHILE OBSERVING ANY CHANGE.

AS A FOLLOW-ON TO STICKING THE TONGUE OUT (WITHOUT PULLING THE HEAD BACK OR HOLDING THE BREATH) — ASK YOUR PUPIL TO BRING THE KNUCKLES OF BOTH HANDS — SLOWLY — TO REST ON THE SIDES OF THE LOWER RIBS...

THEN — DIRECTING THE TIP OF THE TONGUE TO THE TOP (OR BACK) OF THE LOWER TEETH, AND THE JAW AWAY FROM RESTING ON THE THROAT, THINK OF SOMETHING THAT MAKES YOU SMILE, AND WHISPER "AH"...

NOW BRING YOUR PUPIL'S ATTENTION TO THE RIB MOVEMENT AS THE AIR IS EXHALED — AND THEN — AS A RESULT OF EXHALATION — THE MOVEMENT OF THE RIBS ON INHALATION.

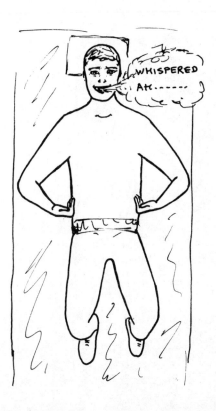

WHISPERED AH......

· ARMS ABOVE YOUR HEAD (SEPARATELY).

THE PRIMARY THING IN THIS ACTIVITY
IS TO MAINTAIN YOUR HEAD – NECK –
BACK RELATIONSHIP, AND YOUR
DIRECTIONS (STIMULUS) TO GO UP...

SO – WHILE STANDING – POINT YOUR
FINGERS TO THE FLOOR...
THEN ROTATE YOUR THUMB AROUND
THE AXIS OF YOUR LITTLE FINGER –
AND THEREBY TURN YOUR HAND INTO
THE ANATOMICAL POSITION...

NOW – BENDING AT THE ELBOW AND
POINTING OR DIRECTING IT TOWARDS
THE FLOOR – RAISE YOUR HAND TO
FACE THE SHOULDER ---

THEN – POINTING YOUR FINGERS TO
THE CEILING – SLOWLY BRING YOUR
HAND ABOVE YOUR HEAD...
AS YOU MOVE (HALF WAY UP) – TURN
YOUR HAND SO THAT YOUR THUMB IS
FACING BEHIND YOU...

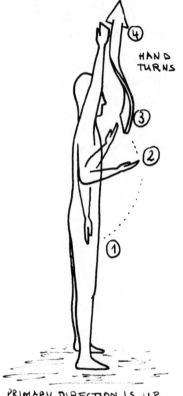

HAND TURNS

PRIMARY DIRECTION IS UP.

BRING YOUR ARM DOWN BY YOUR SIDE
BY SENDING YOUR ELBOW TOWARDS
THE FLOOR ---

THEN REPEAT THE INSTRUCTIONS ON
THE OTHER SIDE – (NOTICE HOW THE
OPPOSITE SIDE OF YOUR NECK
LENGTHENS WITH YOUR ARM RAISED).

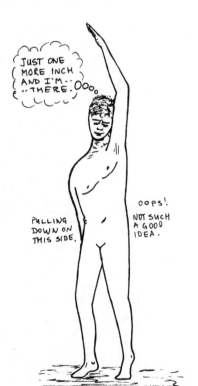

JUST ONE MORE INCH AND I'M ..THERE.. Oooo

PULLING DOWN ON THIS SIDE.

OOPS!. NOT SUCH A GOOD IDEA.

BE VERY CAREFUL THAT YOU DO NOT
IMAGINE YOUR ARM IS LENGTHENING UP
TOWARDS THE CEILING BY PULLING DOWN
ON THE OTHER SIDE, ETC...
THE PURPOSE OF THE ACTIVITY IS NOT
TO SEE HOW HIGH ABOVE YOUR HEAD
YOU CAN LIFT YOUR ARM, BUT RATHER
TO MOVE WITHOUT SHORTENING.

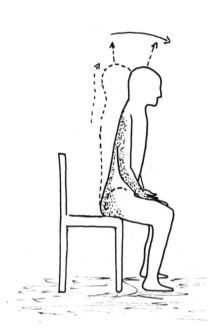

• WHISPERED AH — WHILE FORWARD ON YOUR HANDS.

THE FIRST PART OF THIS GAME CONSISTS OF COMING FORWARD IN THE CHAIR — AND USING YOUR HANDS AND ARMS TO TAKE THE WEIGHT THROUGH INTO THE BACK AND INTO THE SITTING BONES...

SO — WHILE SEATED — SEND YOUR BOTTOM BACK AND DOWN, AND YOUR HEAD FORWARD AND UP...
THEN — WITH YOUR HANDS RESTING PALMS UP ON YOUR LEGS, COME SLIGHTLY FORWARD ON TO YOUR HANDS...
OBSERVE ANY UNNECESSARY ACTIVITY IN THE LEGS ETC...

ONCE FORWARD ON YOUR HANDS LIKE THIS — YOUR RIBS WILL NEED TO BE USED MORE — ALSO THE DIAPHRAGM WILL BE STIMULATED BY THE LENGTHENING OF THE LUMBAR AREA (HIPS BACK AND DOWN) — AND, SINCE YOU HAVE TAKEN THE WEIGHT BY USING THE UPPER LIMBS, YOUR LEGS WILL BE IN A BETTER POSITION TO FREE UP...

ALL THIS ADDS UP TO THE IDEAL SITUATION FOR DOING A WHISPERED AH — SMILE — TIP OF THE TONGUE ETC... AH.....

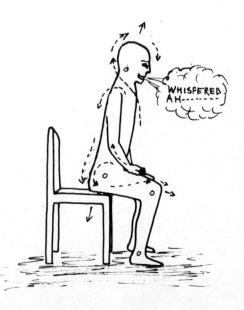

WHISPERED AH...

TERM ONE
SECOND HALF

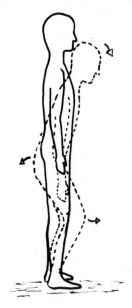

• GOING INTO MONKEY — AND WHISPERED AH.

FIRST OF ALL — WITH YOUR WEIGHT STACKED JOINT UPON JOINT, IN LINE WITH YOUR CENTRE OF BALANCE OVER YOUR HEELS, STIMULATING THE POSITIVE SUPPORTING REFLEX. DIRECT UP AND AWAY FROM THE PULL OF GRAVITY (REHEARSING IT IN YOUR MIND FIRST IS USEFUL)...
AND THEN — WITHOUT STOPPING, OR STRIVING FOR SOME KIND OF PERFECTION — SIMPLY GO AHEAD AND CARRY IT OUT---
HEAD FORWARD — KNEES FORWARD AND HIPS (AND PELVIS) BACK...
GO INTO MONKEY AND SEE WHERE IT TAKES YOU ...

WHILE IN MONKEY — IF YOU WERE GOING TO BEND MECHANICALLY AT THE THE HIP JOINTS, YOUR BOTTOM WOULD TEND TO GO UP (STICK OUT), AND YOUR LEGS TO STRAIGHTEN ETC...
THAT IS — SHORTENING WILL PULL THE KNEES BACK AS THE BODY COMES FORWARD. CLEARLY SHOWING THE IMPORTANCE OF LENGTHENING (FROM THE BACK INTO) THE LEGS AND SENDING THE KNEES FORWARD...

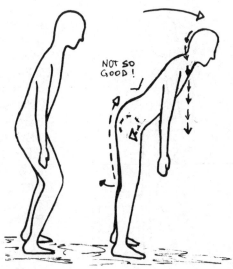

NOT SO GOOD!

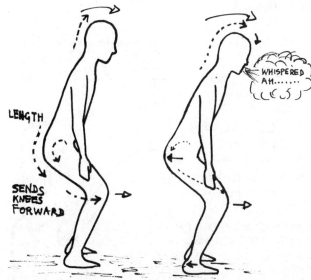

LENGTH

SENDS KNEES FORWARD

WHISPERED AH.......

SO — BEING CAREFUL NOT TO TIGHTEN UNDER YOUR CHIN AND ROOT OF THE TONGUE (THINKING OF YOUR HYOID BONE AND THROAT) AS YOU SET THINGS UP---

PICK ANY EXHALATION (OUT-BREATH), SMILE, TIP OF THE TONGUE TO THE TOP OF THE LOWER TEETH — WHISPER AH...

• HANDS ON THE BACK OF THE CHAIR.

WITH THE BACK OF A CHAIR PLACED
IN FRONT OF YOU – GO INTO MONKEY
TAKING CARE NOT TO PULL DOWN IN
FRONT...
THEN POINTING YOUR FINGERS TO
THE FLOOR – TURN YOUR HANDS INTO
THE ANATOMICAL POSITION...

NOW – BEFORE GOING ANY FURTHER –
REMEMBER THAT MOST OF US WILL
TEND TO USE THE PECTORALS AND
BICEPS TO BEND AT THE ELBOWS
(ESPECIALLY HORSE RIDERS)...

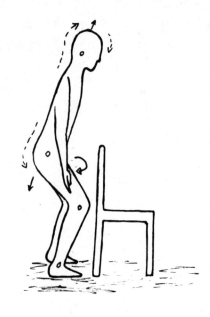

WE WANT TO USE
OUR BRACHIALIS
MUSCLES TO DO
SO –
WITH THIS IN MIND
(DO NOT FORCE OR
RUSH ANYTHING)
AND SENDING YOUR
ELBOWS TOWARDS
THE FLOOR, BRING
BOTH HANDS UP
TO REST ON THE
BACK OF THE
CHAIR...
THINK OF YOUR
SHOULDERS GOING
BACK AND DOWN...

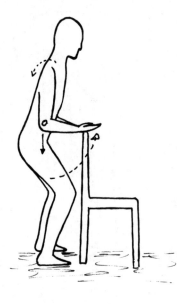

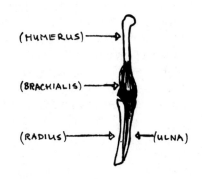

(HUMERUS)

(BRACHIALIS)

(RADIUS)   (ULNA)

F.M. RECOMMENDED THAT
YOU LENGTHEN, OR STRAIGHTEN,
YOUR FINGERS WITH THE OTHER
HAND IF NECESSARY.

IN THIS POSITION, YOUR
ELBOWS WILL EASILY
COME INTO THE SIDE –
THIS, WITH YOUR DIRECTIONS,
HELPS WIDENING:
BUT TOO MUCH ULNAR
DEVIATION WILL HAVE
THE OPPOSITE EFFECT...

NOW, RELEASE YOUR HANDS
FROM SUPINE TO PRONE...
THEN, TAKE THE CHAIR BETWEEN
YOUR FINGERS AND THUMB...
NOW, PULL TO THE ELBOWS, ETC..

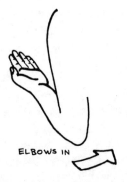

ELBOWS IN

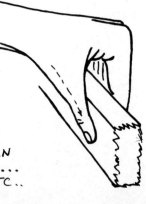

• HANDS ON THE PUPIL'S SHOULDERS — AND ROCKING THE PUPIL.

IN THIS PROCEDURE, THE PUPIL IS SITTING SIDEWAYS ON A CHAIR (WITH THE BACK OF THE CHAIR TO THE SIDE) ---
IN THE SAME WAY AS FOR HANDS ON THE BACK OF A CHAIR — GO INTO MONKEY AT THE PUPIL'S BACK ---
THEN — POINTING YOUR FINGERS TO THE FLOOR — TURN YOUR HANDS INTO THE ANATOMICAL POSITION, AND, SENDING YOUR ELBOWS TOWARDS THE FLOOR, BRING YOUR HANDS UP TO REST (PALMS UP) ON EITHER SHOULDER ---
WITH YOUR ELBOWS GOING INTO THE SIDES — AND WIDENING ACROSS THE UPPER ARMS, CHEST AND BACK — TURN YOUR HANDS SO THAT THE HEELS OF YOUR HANDS COME INTO CONTACT WITH THE SHOULDERS ---

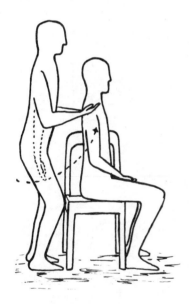

WE USE THE HEELS OF OUR HANDS IN THE SAME WAY AS WE USE THE HEELS OF OUR FEET.
FIRST - ESTABLISH GOOD CONTACT — WITHOUT ANY UNDUE EFFORT — AND THEN LENGTHEN AWAY FROM THE HANDS...
THEN - IMAGINE IT WERE POSSIBLE TO LIFT THE PUPIL OUT OF THE CHAIR SIMPLY BY DIRECTING...

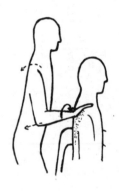

NOW, COME INTO STANDING, AND GENTLY TAKE YOUR HANDS AWAY.

ONCE AGAIN — GO INTO MONKEY AND REPEAT THE PREVIOUS INSTRUCTIONS ---
BUT THIS TIME — GENTLY ROCK YOUR PUPIL BACK AND FORTH OVER THE SITTING BONES.

THERE ARE TWO WAYS TO APPROACH THIS, THE FIRST, USING YOUR ARMS ONLY AND THE SECOND, BY COMING A LITTLE MORE ON TO YOUR HEELS TO ROCK THE PUPIL BACK, AND BY SENDING YOUR KNEES FORWARD TO ROCK FORWARD.

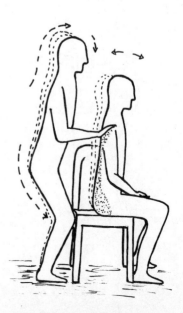

• LIFTING • WITHOUT TIGHTENING THE BICEPS •

STANDING IN FRONT OF A TEACHING TABLE — GO INTO MONKEY —
AND THEN — AS WITH HANDS ON THE BACK OF A CHAIR — BRING
YOUR HANDS UP TO REST (PALMS UP) ON THE TABLE...

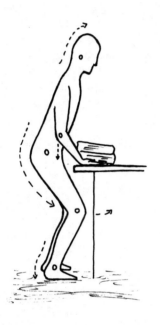

NOW — HAVE SOMEONE
PLACE A NUMBER OF
TELEPHONE BOOKS ON
YOUR HANDS (NOT TOO
HEAVY)...

THEN — SENDING YOUR
ELBOWS TOWARDS THE
FLOOR — GO INTO A
SLIGHTLY DEEPER
MONKEY (BY SENDING
YOUR KNEES FORWARD),
WHILE GRADUALLY
TAKING THE WEIGHT
INTO YOUR BACK —
AND THROUGH ONTO
YOUR HEELS ...

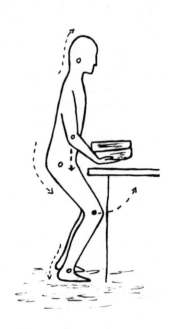

CONTINUE SENDING YOUR
ELBOWS TOWARDS THE
FLOOR — AND, AS YOU
MOVE INTO VERTICAL,
YOUR ELBOWS WILL
ALSO MOVE BACK,
BRINGING THE BOOKS
CLOSER TO YOUR
CHEST...

NOW YOU ARE STANDING —
ALLOW THE WEIGHT OF
THE BOOKS TO BE TAKEN
THROUGH YOUR HEELS,
AND SEND YOUR HEAD
FORWARD AND UP — AND
YOUR BOTTOM BACK AND
DOWN.

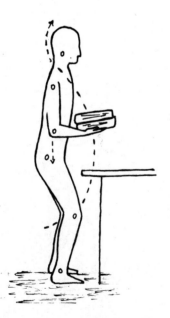

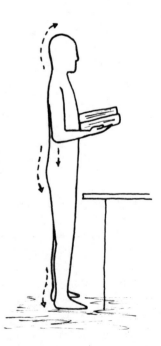

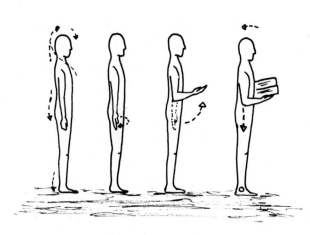

• CARRYING A WEIGHT – WALKING.

WHILE STANDING – POINT YOUR
FINGERS TO THE FLOOR…
THEN – TURN YOUR HANDS INTO
THE ANATOMICAL POSITION…
SENDING YOUR ELBOWS TO THE
FLOOR – BEND AT THE ELBOWS,
AND RAISE BOTH HANDS…
NOW – HAVE SOME TELEPHONE
BOOKS (NOT TOO HEAVY) –
PLACED ON YOUR HANDS, AND,
AS YOU TAKE THE WEIGHT,
SEND YOUR ELBOWS TOWARDS
THE FLOOR, AND GENTLY COME
BACK ON TO YOUR HEELS IN
ORDER TO ADJUST FOR THE
EXTRA WEIGHT TO THE FRONT
OF YOUR BODY…

AT THIS POINT – MAINTAINING THE
FREEDOM IN YOUR ANKLES –
COME BACK A LITTLE (OFF
BALANCE) AND TAKE A STEP
BACKWARDS…
WITH YOUR WEIGHT NOW MORE
ON THE BACK HEEL THAN ON
THE FRONT – THINK OF MOVING
YOUR WEIGHT FORWARD, AND,
AS YOUR HEAD COMES (FORWARD
AND UP) OVER THE FRONT HEEL –
FOLLOW THROUGH WITH THE
BACK LEG INTO WALKING…

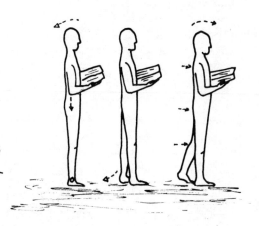

STAGE TWO OF THIS ACTIVITY TAKES
US INTO WALKING – AS ABOVE – BUT
ALSO INVOLVES TURNING ON THE
FORWARD LEG.

SO – AS YOU BRING YOUR WEIGHT OVER
AND ON TO THE FRONT HEEL – LOOK
AND TURN TO THE SAME SIDE, AND
THEN BEND THAT KNEE AS IF YOU
WERE LOWERING A TRAY TO THE
LEVEL OF SOMEONE SEATED…
NOW – COME BACK TO THE START,
AND REPEAT ON THE OTHER SIDE…
THEN – TURNING AND BENDING ON EACH
STEP FORWARD – WALK ON.

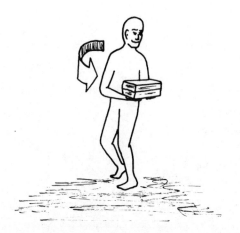

•CRAWLING – AND WHISPERED AH.

CRAWLING IS BEST BEGUN BY GENTLY ROCKING FORWARDS BACKWARDS – WITH THE HEAD LEADING AND THE BODY FOLLOWING AFTER IT...

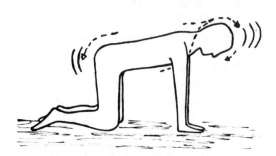

THEN – ALLOW THE PELVIS TO GO IN THE OPPOSITE DIRECTION TO THE HEAD, AND FOLLOW IT – BY ROCKING BACKWARDS – (WHILE CONTINUING TO SEND THE HEAD IN THE OTHER DIRECTION)...

NOW – AS YOU ROCK FORWARD – LOOK AT ONE HAND (TURNING YOUR HEAD AT THE SAME TIME)...
THEN – ALLOW YOUR LEG (OTHER SIDE) TO COME FORWARD AND THUS PROVIDE THE SUPPORT FOR LOCOMOTION...
FOLLOW THIS WITH THE HAND YOU ARE LOOKING AT – WHILE AT THE SAME TIME SWITCHING YOUR ATTENTION TO THE OTHER HAND – YOU ARE NOW CRAWLING FORWARD.

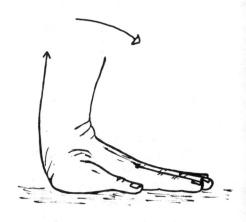

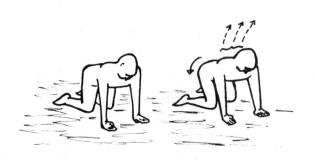

EVERY TIME YOU ROCK FORWARD, YOU HYPER-EXTEND YOUR WRISTS, SO TAKE CARE NOT TO OVERDO IT...
ALSO – TOO MUCH WEIGHT FORWARD CAN PULL YOU DOWN IN FRONT – IN WHICH CASE – COME BACK A BIT...

THE TEACHER MAY PLACE A HAND UNDER YOUR FOREHEAD FOR SUPPORT, AND TO HELP LIFT THE "COLLAR"...
ON HORSES THE CARRIAGE OF THE HEAD AND NECK AFFECTS THE DISTRIBUTION OF WEIGHT ON THE LEGS, RAISING THE NECK, COMING BACK A LITTLE ON TO THE HIND LEGS (AS WE WOULD WHEN ROCKING BACKWARDS) HELPS TO AVOID PULLING THE "COLLAR" DOWN.
TRY A WHISPERED AH AS THE HAND COMES TO THE GROUND... (KNEE FORWARD – IN-BREATH, HAND FORWARD – OUT BREATH... IN MUCH THE SAME WAY AS HORSES DO).

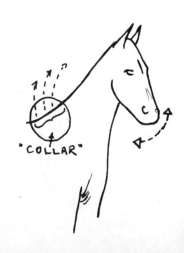

"COLLAR"

· SQUATTING – WITH AID OF A CHAIR.

STANDING IN FRONT OF A CHAIR – ALLOWING YOUR HEELS TO
TO TAKE YOUR WEIGHT – YOUR HEAD TO GO FORWARD AND UP –
AND YOUR HIPS (PELVIS) TO GO BACK AND DOWN OVER FREED
ANKLE AND KNEE JOINTS ...
NOW – HEAD AND KNEES FORWARD, AND HIPS BACK – GO INTO
MONKEY ...
FOLLOW THROUGH INTO A DEEPER MONKEY, ALLOWING YOUR
HIPS BACK AND DOWN TO HELP SEND YOUR KNEES FURTHER
FORWARD, THEN THE HEELS WILL NOT BE PULLED OFF THE FLOOR.
AS YOU PROCEED DEEPER, PLACE BOTH HANDS ON THE CHAIR
TO ACT AS SECURITY AND SUPPORT ...

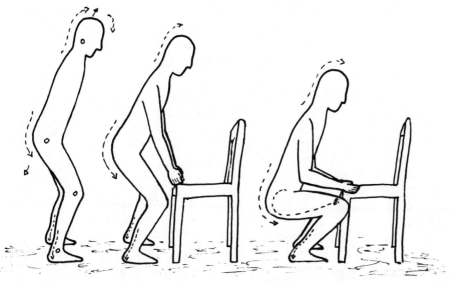

PULLING TO THE ELBOWS – (WIDTH ACROSS THE
UPPER CHEST AND ARMS) – COME FORWARD
A LITTLE, AND AT THE SAME TIME – DROP
YOUR BOTTOM WHILE SENDING YOUR HEAD
IN THE OPPOSITE DIRECTION ...
DO NOT STAY IN SQUAT. INSTEAD, RETURN
TO UPRIGHT IN ONE FLOWING MOVEMENT.

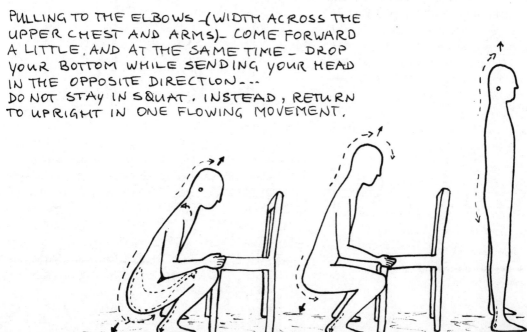

• WALKING UP STAIRS .

STANDING – WITH YOUR WEIGHT EVENLY DISTRIBUTED ON BOTH HEELS –
GRADUALLY BEND ONE FOOT AT THE JOINT OF THE BIG TOE – WHILE
ALLOWING THE WEIGHT OF THAT SIDE TO BE TAKEN ON THE BALL OF
THE FOOT – BENDING AT THE KNEE,
NOW BRING YOUR HEEL BACK TO THE FLOOR, AND REPEAT ON THE OTHER SIDE.

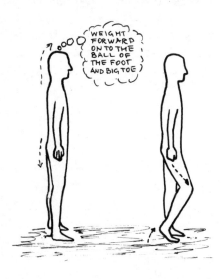

HAVING COMPLETED THE ABOVE
INSTRUCTIONS – THIS TIME GO
AS FAR AS, "BEND THE FOOT AT
THE BIG TOE"...
THEN – FLICK THAT FOOT
FORWARD – BRINGING IT TO IN
FRONT OF THE OTHER...
NOW – BRING IT BACK TO WHERE
YOU STARTED – AND REPEAT
ON THE OTHER SIDE.

WHEN GOING UP STAIRS – WE
USUALLY GO FORWARD ON TO
THE RAISED FOOT AND THEN
STRAIGHTEN IT PULLING
DOWN IN THE PROCESS...

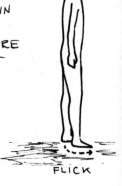

FLICK

NOW – PLACE A STEP, OR
SOME TELEPHONE BOOKS,
IN FRONT OF YOU – OR –
STAND AT THE FOOT OF
THE STAIRS ...
AND, AT THE POINT WHERE
YOU BEND AT THE BIG
TOE, FLICK YOUR FOOT
FORWARD AND UP ON
TO THE STEP IN FRONT
(INCLUDING THE HEEL)...

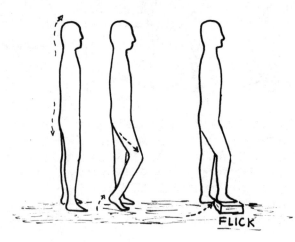

FLICK

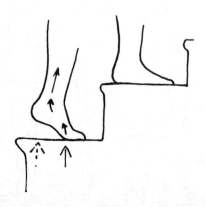

NOW – WITH THE BACK (OR LOWER)
FOOT... BRING THE WEIGHT FORWARD
ON TO THE JOINT OF THE BIG TOE (THUS
BENDING THE FOOT) ... AND THEN – PUSH
FROM THERE TO BRING THAT FOOT UP, TO
BESIDE THE OTHER ONE ...
CONTINUE ON UP THE STAIRS – AIMING
OR DIRECTING YOUR HEAD TOWARDS THE
TOP OF THE STAIRS.

PART THREE

CONTINUED

TERM TWO
FIRST HALF

. TAKING A PUPIL'S ARM AND HAND.

FIRST_ POSITION YOURSELF TO THE SIDE OF THE SEATED PUPIL...
THEN_GO INTO MONKEY (CHECKING YOUR DIRECTIONS THROUGHOUT)...
NOW_ PRESUMING THAT THE PUPIL'S HANDS ARE RESTING (PALMS UP)
ON HIS OR HER LEGS_ PLACE YOUR STRAIGHTENED FINGERS (AS
IN HANDS ON THE BACK OF A CHAIR) IN THE PALM OF YOUR PUPIL'S
HAND...

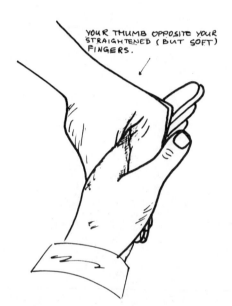

YOUR THUMB OPPOSITE YOUR
STRAIGHTENED (BUT SOFT)
FINGERS.

TAKE CARE NOT TO GRAB THE HAND_
RISKING A REACTION IN YOUR PUPIL,
NOT TO MENTION WHAT IT WOULD DO
TO YOU. INSTEAD, BRING YOUR
THUMB AROUND TO THE BACK OF
THE PUPIL'S HAND (AS IF IT WERE
THE RAIL OF A CHAIR) AND OPPOSITE
YOUR STRAIGHTENED FINGERS...

REMEMBER THAT WHEN YOU MOVE THE
HAND AND ARM _ THE CHEST WILL
AUTOMATICALLY BE INVOLVED _
SINCE THE MUSCLES OF THE
SHOULDER GIRDLE AFFECT THE
INTERCOSTALS...

NOW_ PLACE YOUR OTHER HAND UNDER THE
PUPIL'S ARM _ BETWEEN THE RIBS (AT THE
BACK OF YOUR HAND) AND THE ARM OR
BICEPS (AT THE PALM OF YOUR HAND).
IT IS VERY EASY TO PULL OR PUSH YOUR
PUPIL, IF THE SHOULDER ARE TIGHT...SO...

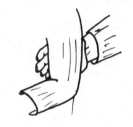

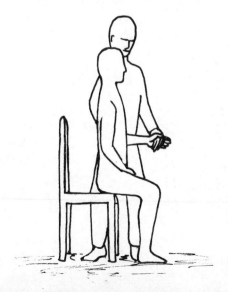

IN ORDER TO GIVE CLEAR DIRECTIONS,
ASK YOUR PUPIL TO USE THE EYES
(NOT TO STARE), AND TO ALLOW THEIR
SITTING BONES TO TAKE THEIR
WEIGHT THROUGH TO THE CHAIR_
(IT IS WHAT HAPPENS IN THE TRUNK
THAT ENCOURAGES THE HEAD TO GO
FORWARD AND UP)...

NOW_TAKE THE HAND AND ARM OUT
IN FRONT OF THE PUPIL (AS IF TO
PLACE IT ON THE BACK OF A CHAIR).
LENGTHENING AND WIDENING AS YOU
GO.

· HANDS ON THE BACK OF A CHAIR — ALTERNATIVE APPROACH.

AS USUAL — BEGIN WITH YOUR HANDS DOWN BY YOUR SIDES (IN THIS CASE WHILE SEATED)....
THEN — WITH POINTING FINGERS — TURN YOUR HANDS—THUMBS AROUND LITTLE FINGERS — INTO THE ANATOMICAL POSITION...

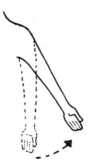 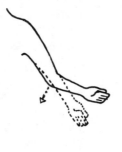 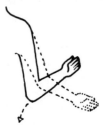

NOW — SLOWLY BRING ONE ARM OUT TO THE SIDE (STILL POINTING)...
THEN — HALF WAY UP — BEGIN TO SEND YOUR ELBOW TOWARDS THE FLOOR...
AND — BENDING AT THE ELBOW — BRING YOUR UPPER ARM INTO THE SIDE...
FINALLY — BRING YOUR HAND AROUND TO (POINTING) IN FRONT OF YOU...

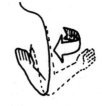

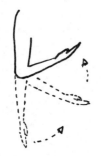

YOU ARE NOW IN A POSITION TO PLACE YOUR HAND ON THE BACK OF THE CHAIR IN FRONT OF YOU ...
REPEAT WITH THE OTHER HAND — ETC ...
THE OTHER APPROACH BASICALLY INVOLVES BENDING AT THE ELBOWS, AND — SENDING YOUR ELBOWS TOWARDS THE FLOOR — RAISING YOUR HANDS.

THIS IS USUALLY HOW WE BRING THE HAND UP..

ALLOWING YOUR BOTTOM TO GO INTO, OR FALL TOWARDS, THE CHAIR — SEND YOUR HEAD FORWARD AND UP — ROCKING YOURSELF SLIGHTLY FORWARD ON YOUR SITTING BONES...
CAREFUL THOUGH — WE ALL HAVE A TENDENCY TO PULL OUR HEADS BACK AS WE MOVE FORWARD.

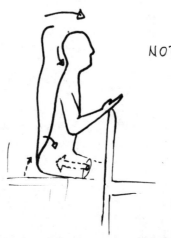

NOT GOOD!

NO POINT IN CONTINUING. IF THIS TAKES PLACE ...
BEGIN AGAIN.

• ARMS ABOVE YOUR HEAD — ONE AFTER THE OTHER — REPEATING.

WHILE SEATED IN A CHAIR — WE WANT OUR SITTING BONES TO
TAKE OUR WEIGHT—VERTICALLY STACKED (IN BALANCE) ABOVE
THEM — SO THAT OUR BACKS CAN LENGTHEN AND WIDEN FROM THAT
BASE — AND OUR NECKS TO BE FREE, SO THE HEAD CAN GO
FORWARD AND UP...

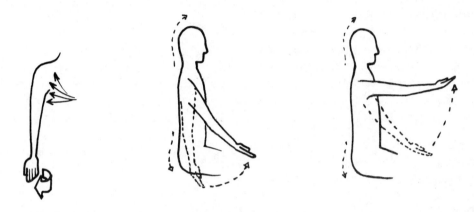

THEN — POINTING YOUR FINGERS TO THE
FLOOR — TURN YOUR HANDS INTO THE
ANATOMICAL POSITION...
NOW — BRING YOUR HAND AND ARM UP TO
SHOULDER LEVEL IN FRONT OF YOU...
FOLLOWING THIS — BRING YOUR HAND
OUT TO THE SIDE...
AND THEN — UP TO ABOVE YOUR HEAD...
FINALLY — LOWER YOUR HAND AND ARM
IN FRONT OF YOU — AND BACK TO THE SIDE...
NOW — REPEAT ON THE OTHER SIDE...

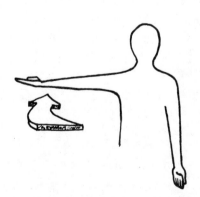
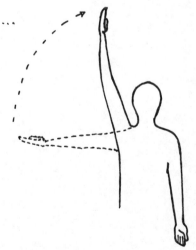

AT THIS STAGE OF THE ACTIVITY, BEGIN WITH ONE HAND AND
ARM, AND AS YOU ARE COMPLETING THE MOVEMENT, START WITH
THE OTHER... UNTIL IT BECOMES ONE FLOWING MOVEMENT.

· WHISPERED AH – WITH YOUR BACK CLOSE TO THE WALL.

THE IDEA OF STANDING WITH YOUR BACK CLOSE TO THE WALL,
IS FOR NO OTHER REASON THAN TO PROVIDE YOU WITH ENOUGH
CONFIDENCE TO COME BACK A LITTLE MORE ON TO YOUR HEELS
WITHOUT THE FEAR OF FALLING BACKWARDS...
THEREBY LIMITING THE EFFECTS OF UNNECESSARY TENSION ON
THE POSTURAL REFLEXES – AND THEN ALLOWING THE BREATHING TO
OPERATE MORE FREELY...

SO– STANDING IN A MANNER DESCRIBED ABOVE – WITH YOUR
WEIGHT BEING TAKEN LARGELY THROUGH THE HEELS, YOUR
HEAD GOING FORWARD AND UP (ACTING AS A BALANCER) AND
YOUR BOTTOM GOING BACK AND DOWN (NOT CLENCHED)···
GENTLY ROCK OR HINGE BACKWARDS ON YOUR ANKLES AND
HEELS (LIKE THE LID OF A BOX – ALL ONE PIECE)···
NOW– THE TIP OF THE TONGUE TO THE TOP OF THE LOWER
TEETH – THINK OF SOMETHING THAT MAKES YOU SMILE – ALLOW THE
JAW TO DROP AND WHISPER AH...

THE NEXT TIME – DO IT IN FRONT OF A CHAIR INSTEAD.

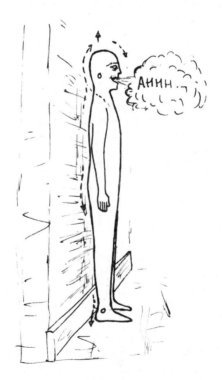

IN VOICE WORK, NOT ENOUGH ATTENTION IS PAID TO THE
DIRECTION TO COME BACK ONTO THE HEELS, WITH THE
RESULT, PEOPLE END UP FORWARD OVER THE TOES, AND
HAVING TO FORCE THE BREATHING.

· GOING UP STAIRS .

BEGIN BY STANDING AT THE FOOT OF THE STAIRS (OR STEPS)
THEN — TO PROVIDE THE CONDITIONS FAVOURABLE FOR
LENGTHENING AND WIDENING — ALLOW YOUR WEIGHT TO BE
TAKEN THROUGH AND INTO THE FLOOR, BY COMING INTO
BALANCE OVER YOUR HEELS...
NOW — THINKING OF THE WEIGHT AROUND THE OUTSIDES OF THE
FEET — SEND ONE KNEE FORWARD WHILE BENDING AT THE BALL
OF THAT FOOT (AT BIG TOE JOINT...
AND THEN — FLICK YOUR FOOT FORWARD AND UP ON TO THE STEP
IN FRONT — (BE CAREFUL NOT TO SHIFT YOUR PELVIS OUT TO THE
OPPOSITE SIDE IN THE PROCESS)...

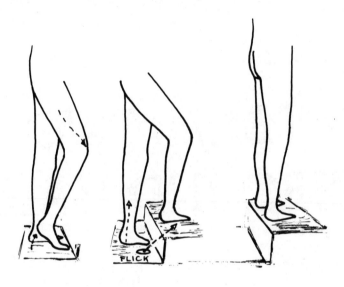

FLICK

NOW — DIRECTING FROM THE BACK FOOT — BRING YOUR WEIGHT
AROUND THE OUTSIDE (OF THE SAME FOOT) AND ON TO THE
BIG TOE JOINT ...
THEN, BENDING AT THE TOES , 'PUSH WITH THE BACK FOOT
TO BRING IT UP TO BESIDE THE OTHER ONE...

CONTINUE ON UP THE STAIRS IN A FLOWING MANNER —
BEING CAREFUL NOT TO PULL DOWN IN FRONT AS YOU GO.

TERM TWO
SECOND HALF

• MOVING YOUR EYES — WITHOUT MOVING
YOUR HEAD.

WHILE SEATED — ALLOW YOUR WEIGHT TO BE
TAKEN INTO THE CHAIR BY BALANCING
OVER YOUR SITTING-BONES ...
THEN — WHEN YOU ARE HAPPY WITH YOUR
DIRECTIONS — POINT YOUR FINGERS
TOWARDS THE FLOOR AND OPEN BOTH
HANDS ...
NOW — TURN THEM (THUMBS AROUND THE
LITTLE FINGERS) INTO THE ANATOMICAL
POSITION ...
AND THEN — ALLOWING YOUR SHOULDERS
TO REST BACK AND DOWN ON THE
RIB CAGE — BRING YOUR FINGERS UP
TO BEHIND THE JAW, AND UNDER THE
EARS ...
FINALLY — NOD YOUR HEAD TO CHECK THAT
YOU ARE NOT HOLDING ON ...

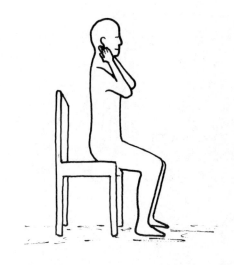

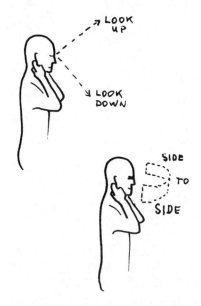

LOOK
UP

LOOK
DOWN

SIDE
TO
SIDE

HAVING COMPLETED THE
INSTRUCTIONS SO FAR — AND
USING YOUR FINGERS TO
MONITOR INVOLUNTARY HEAD
MOVEMENT ---

LOOK UP TO THE CEILING —
OBSERVING ANY ACTIVITY AS
A RESULT OF THE EYE
MOVEMENT ...
THEN — LOOK DOWN TOWARDS
THE FLOOR, AND ONCE AGAIN,
OBSERVE ...
NEXT — LOOK TO THE LEFT.
AND FINALLY — LOOK TO THE
RIGHT.

IF THE PUPIL HOLDS ON IN THE
NECK IN AN ATTEMPT TO
FORCE THE HEAD NOT TO MOVE,
THEN DO NOT CONTINUE ---

CAREFUL NOT TO LIFT THE
SHOULDERS AS YOU BRING
YOUR HANDS UP ...
OR LOWER YOUR HEAD
TOWARDS THE HANDS.

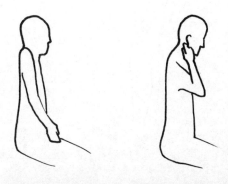

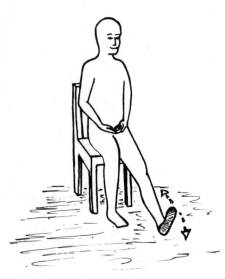

• FREEING THE ANKLES.

SEATED IN A CHAIR — THINK OF YOUR
HEEL (EITHER HEEL) POINTING AWAY
FROM YOU...
THEN SEND THAT FOOT FORWARD AND
STRAIGHTEN YOUR LEG IN THE
PROCESS...
AND THEN — ONCE SATISFIED YOU ARE
NOT HOLDING ON IN YOUR LEG (OR
ANYWHERE ELSE FOR THAT MATTER)
POINT YOUR TOES (TO THE SKY), AND
AT THE SAME TIME FLEX YOUR
FOOT — AND THEN, EXTEND IT...

YOU MAY FIND IT NECESSARY TO
REMOVE YOUR SHOE, AS ITS HEEL
MAY FORCE YOU TO PUSH...

TAKE YOUR TIME, AND BE CAREFUL
NOT TO TIGHTEN IN THE LEGS AND
PULL DOWN...
NOW — THINKING OF YOUR LITTLE TOE —
MOVE YOUR FOOT FROM SIDE TO
SIDE...
THEN REPEAT, THINKING OF THE BIG TOE....
AND FINALLY — DESCRIBE A CIRCLE WITH
YOUR LITTLE TOE (DIRECT FROM THE
HEEL) — FIRST TO THE RIGHT, THEN LEFT...
AND AGAIN — THIS TIME WITH THE BIG TOE.

TO THE RIGHT
THINKING OF THE
LITTLE TOE - THEN
TO THE LEFT

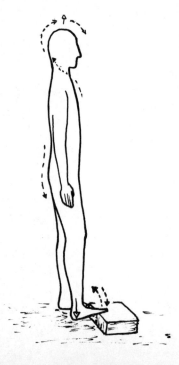

AND NOW..WHILE STANDING .. WITH
A TELEPHONE BOOK PLACED CLOSE
TO ONE FOOT...
BRING YOUR TOES UP TO REST ON
THE BOOK — LEAVING THE HEEL OF
THAT FOOT ON THE FLOOR...
THEN — DIRECTING YOUR HEEL INTO
THE FLOOR — RAISE YOUR TOES OFF
THE BOOK, AND BACK AGAIN.

WITH ALL OF THESE ACTIVITIES IT IS
TAKEN FOR GRANTED YOU REPEAT
THEM ON THE OTHER SIDE...

BUT WITH THE SEATED ACTIVITIES —
YOU FINALLY REPEAT THE GAMES
WITH BOTH LEGS OUT IN FRONT,

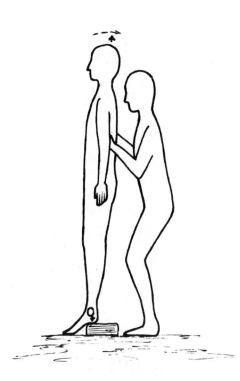

· FREEING THE ANKLES _ (CONTINUED)

STANDING _ THIS TIME WITH YOUR
HEELS ON THE TELEPHONE BOOKS,
(ONE UNDER EACH HEEL), AND YOUR
TOES ON THE FLOOR ...

WITH THE "SUPPORT OF A TEACHER
BEHIND _ GENTLY COME BACK INTO
HIS OR HER HANDS, WHILE AT THE
SAME TIME ALLOWING YOUR
TOES TO REMAIN RESTING ON THE
FLOOR ...
THIS IS ONLY POSSIBLE WHEN THE
ANKLES ARE FREE ENOUGH.

ONCE AGAIN _ STANDING WITH
YOUR HEELS ON THE BOOKS,
AND YOUR TOES ON THE
FLOOR ...

COME BACK GENTLY INTO THE
TEACHER'S HANDS _ AND WITH
FREE ANKLES _ LEAVE YOUR
TOES ON THE FLOOR ...

NOW _ MAKING SURE YOU DO
NOT GRIP OR PULL DOWN _
BRING YOUR TOES (BOTH FEET)
OFF THE FLOOR WHILE
POINTING THEM AT THE SAME
TIME.

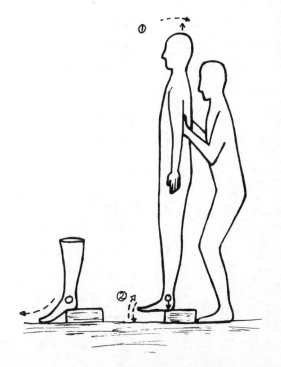

• GOING DOWN STAIRS.

STANDING ON TELEPHONE
BOOKS - OR A PLATFORM
WITH ENOUGH ROOM FOR
BOTH FEET (HEELS AND
TOES)...

COME INTO BALANCE OVER
BOTH HEELS SO THAT
YOUR HEAD CAN GO
FORWARD AND UP - YOUR
SHOULDERS CAN GO BACK
AND DOWN - AND YOUR
BOTTOM CAN ALSO DO THE
SAME - SO THAT YOUR
BACK CAN LENGTHEN AND
WIDEN...

NOW - SIMPLY POINT TOWARDS
THE FLOOR WITH YOUR BIG
TOE (FOR EXAMPLE - THE
RIGHT TOE), SO THAT YOU
ARE LEADING WITH THAT
TOE ...

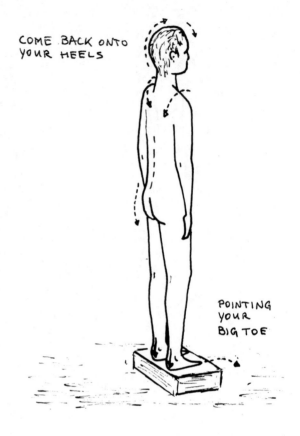

COME BACK ONTO
YOUR HEELS

POINTING
YOUR
BIG TOE

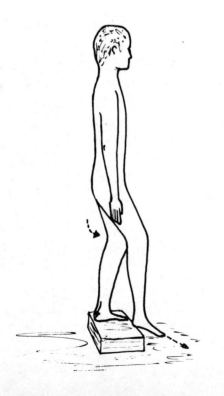

THEN - TRANSFERRING SOME
OF YOUR ATTENTION ON TO THE
LEFT HEEL - GENTLY ALLOW
YOUR WEIGHT TO TRANSFER
WHILE AVOIDING ANY SHIFT
OF THE PELVIS OUT TO THE
SIDE...
THEN - STILL POINTING WITH
THE BIG TOE OF THE RIGHT
FOOT - ALLOW YOUR LEFT
KNEE TO BEND WHILE YOU
FOLLOW THROUGH WITH THE
RIGHT FOOT ON TO THE STEP
BELOW...

NOW - IF AT THE TOP OF THE
STAIRS - CONTINUE INTO A
FLOWING MOVEMENT - USING
THE BIG TOES TO LEAD...
(CAREFUL NOT TO PULL DOWN).

• ARMS - A PREPARATION FOR WRITING.

SITTING IN BALANCE OVER YOUR SITTING BONES, WITH YOUR ARMS
DOWN BY YOUR SIDE (IN THE ANATOMICAL POSITION) ---
POINT YOUR FINGERS TOWARDS THE FLOOR - AS THOUGH IT WERE
POSSIBLE TO TOUCH THE GROUND WITH THE TIPS ...
NOW - GRADUALLY BRING BOTH HANDS OUT AND UP TO THE SIDE ---

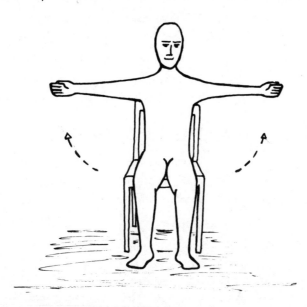

THEN - SENDING YOUR ELBOWS TOWARDS THE FLOOR - BEND YOUR
ARMS, SO THAT YOUR THUMBS COME TOWARDS THE SHOULDERS ...
AND THEN - BRING THE PALMS OF YOUR HANDS AROUND TO REST ON
YOUR CHEST ...
NOW - REVERSE THE PROCEDURE BY BRINGING YOUR HANDS AND
ARMS BACK OUT TO THE SIDE AND FINALLY DOWN TO THE SIDE.

THROUGHOUT THE ACTIVITIES THINK OF THE SHOULDERS GOING
BACK AND DOWN (SHOULDER BLADES TOWARDS THE SITTING-BONES).

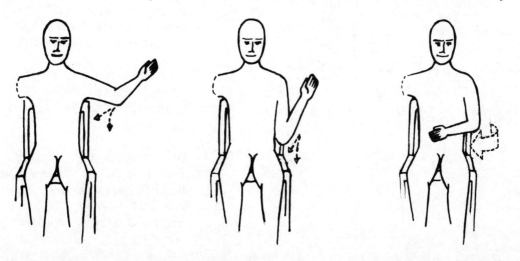

- PREPARATION FOR WRITING.

FOLLOW THE PREVIOUS INSTRUCTIONS UP TO (BUT NOT INCLUDING)
RESTING YOUR HANDS ON YOUR CHEST...

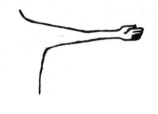 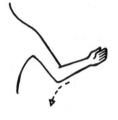 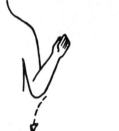 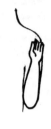

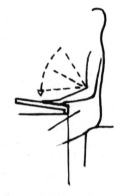

THEN - POINTING YOUR
FINGERS - BRING THE
HAND DOWN TO REST
(PALM DOWN) ON THE
WRITING SURFACE...

NOW - ROTATE YOUR
THUMB AROUND THE
LITTLE FINGER AXIS
NOT UNLIKE THE LID
OF A BOX WITH THE
HINGE ON THE LITTLE
FINGER ...
PALM UP - PALM DOWN -
AND SO ON ...

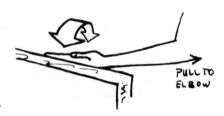

PULL TO
ELBOW

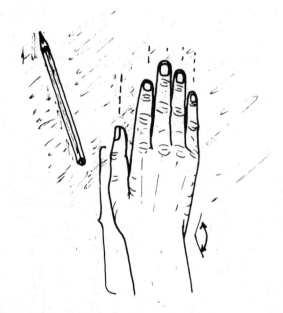

WITH BOTH HANDS ON THE
WRITING SURFACE - USE
THE NON-WRITING HAND TO
STABLISE THE PAPER ...

DO NOT FORGET TO PULL
TO THE ELBOWS -
SHOULDERS BACK AND
DOWN ETC..

THEN - THINK OF POINTING
THE FINGERS AWAY - WITH
ULNAR DEVIATION
ALLOWING THE THUMB TO
EXTEND AWAY ALSO.

· WRITING .

IDEALLY - WE WANT AS MUCH FREEDOM THROUGHOUT THE WHOLE
SYSTEM AS POSSIBLE , SO THAT WE CAN CONFINE THE "DOING" TO
THE MOVEMENT OF THE PEN ...
WHEN WE COME FORWARD FROM THE HIPS - WE CAN DIRECT
LENGTHEN AWAY, OR UP, FROM THE NONWRITING HAND, WHILE AT
THE SAME TIME USING IT AS A SUPPORT, THUS ALLOWING THE
WRITING HAND TO BE USED EXCLUSIVELY FOR WRITING ...
WHEN THE WRITING HAND IS FREE , SO TOO WILL BE THE   DER -
AND NECK ETC ...

MAKE SURE YOUR ELBOWS CLEAR THE WORKING SURFACE WHEN
ESTABLISHING CHAIR HEIGHT - BUT TAKE CARE - TOO HIGH, AND
PULLING DOWN WILL BE HARD TO RESIST ...
SITTING CLOSE TO THE WORK SURFACE HELPS PREVENT (OR LIMIT)
PULLING DOWN ...

LENGTHEN FROM YOUR BACK TO YOUR FINGER TIPS - AND PULL TO
THE ELBOW (FINGER TIPS AWAY FROM THE ELBOW), WHILE
WIDENING ACROSS THE UPPER BACK AND CHEST (UPPER ARMS).

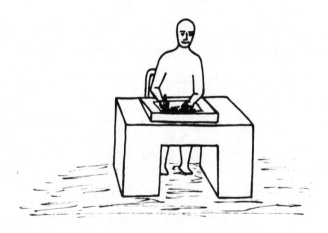

AS THE NERVOUS SYSTEM DEVELOPS , NEUROLOGICAL INHIBITION
ALSO DEVELOPS , WITH THE RESULT THAT EACH STIMULUS
RECEIVED NO LONGER ACTIVATES ALL AVAILABLE MOTOR NERVES,

INHIBITION LIMITS EXTRANEOUS NEUROLOGICAL AND
MUSCULAR ACTIVITY , THUS CLEARING THE WAY FOR
DIRECTION.

•WALKING.

BEGIN BY STANDING WITH BOTH FEET
ACTING LIKE THREE-LEGGED STOOLS,
AND ALLOW YOUR WEIGHT TO BALANCE
OVER YOUR TWO HEELS...
THEN _ THINK OF ONE FOOT _ AND
OBSERVE HOW THE BALANCE (OF WEIGHT)
SHIFTS GRADUALLY ACROSS...
THEN THINK OF THE OTHER FOOT,

NEXT_ ALLOW YOUR
WEIGHT TO COME BACK
A LITTLE MORE OVER
THE HEELS _ AND TO
STIMULATE THE
RESPONSE TO TAKE
A SMALL STEP
BACKWARDS ...

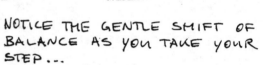

NOTICE THE GENTLE SHIFT OF
BALANCE AS YOU TAKE YOUR
STEP...
AND THEN _ AS YOU SHIFT TO THE
BACK FOOT _ OBSERVE HOW THE
WEIGHT MOVES AWAY FROM THE
FRONT OF THE FRONT FOOT TO
THE HEEL AND THEN AWAY_
THUS FREEING THAT LEG ...

NOW_ THINK OF SENDING YOUR
WEIGHT (BALANCE) OVER ON
TO THE FRONT FOOT...
AND AS YOU MOVE ACROSS_
ALLOW THE BACK LEG TO
SWING FORWARD ---
CONTINUE INTO WALKING...

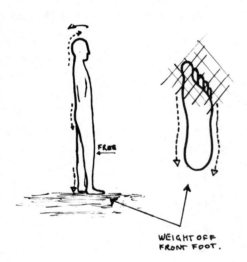

WEIGHT OFF
FRONT FOOT.

AS YOU COME FORWARD ON TO
THE FRONT FOOT _ THE FIRST
PART TO RECEIVE YOUR WEIGHT
WOULD BE THE HEEL _ THEN
THE SIDE _ AND THEN THE BALL
OF THE FOOT (MOVING FORWARD).

DANCERS GENERALLY POINT THE
TOES AND LIFT THE HEEL _ SO
DISALLOWING LENGH _ WHEREAS
IN RUNNING _ THE ANKLES AND FEET
MUST BE FREE (FOR A NATURAL ACTION).

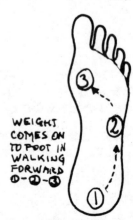

WEIGHT
COMES ON
TO FOOT IN
WALKING
FORWARD
①-②-③

• WHISPERED AH.

WHILE STANDING — BRING YOUR ATTENTION TO THE FLOW OF AIR AS YOU
BREATHE OUT DURING TIDAL (OR QUIET) BREATHING ...
THEN — THINK ABOUT THE DIRECTION IN WHICH IT TRAVELS, THAT IS,
UPWARDS, AND TURNING TO COME OUT YOUR MOUTH ...
NOW — USING THIS UNDERSTANDING TO SEND YOUR HEAD FORWARD
AND UP — GRADUALLY INCREASE THE OUTBREATH, WHILE AT
THE SAME TIME MAKING SURE NOT TO PULL DOWN IN FRONT AS
YOU DO SO ...
NOW — PICK AN OUTBREATH AND DO A WHISPERED AH ---

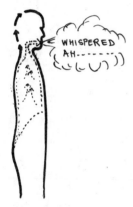

WHISPERED
AH------

BREATHING OUT
TO BREATHE IN

IT IS VERY EASY TO STARE
WHILE DOING WHISPERED
AH'S, SO DO NOT FORGET
THE EYES ...

EVEN LONG AFTER WE
HAVE BEEN HAVING
LESSONS — WE STILL TEND
TO PULL DOWN AS WE
BREATHE OUT, AND THEN
END UP DOING THE IN-
BREATH ...
SO — AFTER EXHALING,
WITHOUT PULLING DOWN,
ALLOW THE IN-BREATH
TO "SPRING" BACK INTO
ACTION, AS A REFLEX
RESPONSE TO THE OUT-
BREATH ...

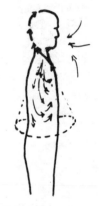

ACHIEVE FULL HEIGHT

BREATHING OUT
TO BREATHE IN

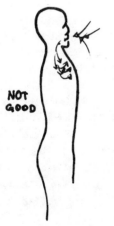

NOT
GOOD

PULLING
DOWN IN
FRONT

IN   FOR OUT.. OOPS!

A LOT OF VOICE USERS TEND
TO THINK THAT IN ORDER TO
FREE UP, AND EXPAND THE
CHEST — IT IS NECESSARY
TO TAKE A DEEP BREATH,
BUT BEFORE YOU EVEN
THINK OF SINGING ETC..
YOU NEED TO ACHIEVE
YOUR FULL HEIGHT ...
IF YOU THEN TRY TO GO
BEYOND THE COMMAND TO
LENGTHEN AND WIDEN, YOU
WILL PULL DOWN IN THE
PROCESS.

• WHISPERED AH, AND STICKING YOUR TONGUE OUT.

STANDING — AND TAKING CARE NOT TO HITCH YOUR SHOULDERS UP — BRING BOTH HANDS UP TO THE LOWER RIBS (OR ABOVE THE ILIAC CREST)..
THEN — PULLING TO THE ELBOWS — ALLOW YOUR SHOULDERS TO GO BACK AND DOWN, WHILE AT THE SAME TIME, COMING UP IN FRONT AS THE HEAD GOES FORWARD AND UP...
NOW — PICK ANY OUTBREATH AND DO A WHISPERED AH...

NOTICE THE TEMPTATION TO TAKE A LITTLE EXTRA AIR IN BEFORE THE AH...
ALTHOUGH NEARLY ALL OF US WILL TEND TO PULL DOWN IN FRONT AS WE BREATHE OUT — USE THE WHISPERED AH TO OBSERVE ANY PULLING DOWN OF THE STERNUM.

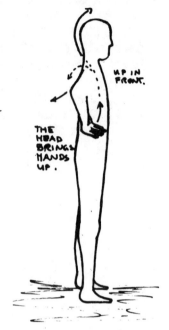

UP IN FRONT.

THE HEAD BRINGS HANDS UP.

OOPS!

OOPS!

AGAIN — WHILE STANDING — IMAGINE YOUR TONGUE COMING ALL THE WAY UP FROM YOUR SYMPHYSIS PUBIS OR PUBIC BONE...
THEN — SLOWLY STICK THE TONGUE OUT — TAKING CARE NOT TO DISTURBE THE BALANCE OF THE HEAD — NECK — BACK RELATIONSHIP.

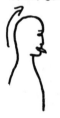

MUCH BETTER.

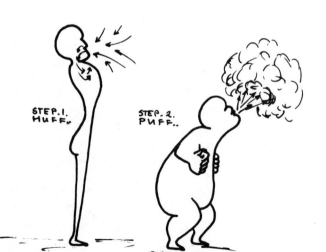

STEP. 1. HUFF.

STEP. 2. PUFF..

A COMMON MISCONCEPTION WITH REGARD TO BREATHING...

"TAKE A DEEP BREATH AND BLOW HARD" — THIS PRODUCES THE BELIEF THAT WE LIFT OURSELVES UP TO BREATHE IN AND AS A RESULT — PULL DOWN TO BREATHE OUT.

PART THREE

CONTINUED

TERM THREE
FIRST HALF

KNEES FORWARD AND AWAY, AND TAKING YOUR WEIGHT THROUGH THE ARMS.

WHILE SEATED_ ALLOW YOUR SITTING BONES TO TAKE YOUR WEIGHT_ AND YOUR HEAD TO ACT AS A BALANCER BY GOING FORWARD AND UP. ... THEN_ COME GRADUALLY FORWARD ON TO YOUR HANDS (PALMS UP, ON YOUR LEGS)....,
STOP AS SOON AS YOU OBSERVE YOUR LEGS TAKING THE WEIGHT...

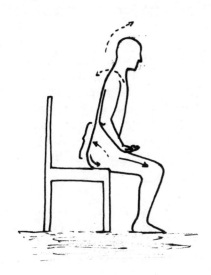

MAKE SURE THE WEIGHT IS BEING TAKEN THROUGH YOUR BACK, AND INTO THE CHAIR VIA YOUR SITTING BONES BY USING YOUR ARMS ONLY.

OTHERWISE YOU RUN THE RISK OF TIGHTENING IN THE LEGS, AND SO, DISTURBING THE BALANCE...

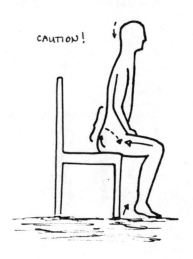

CAUTION!

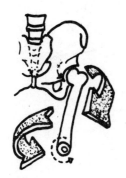

BY NOT USING YOUR LEGS, YOU ALLOW THEM TO MOVE AWAY FROM THE HIP JOINTS ...

THEN_ AS YOU ROCK SLIGHTLY FORWARD, THE HEAD OF THE FEMUR BEING MOVED IN THE ACETABULUM (SOCKET), OPENS THE LEGS (KNEES AWAY FROM EACH- OTHER) ...

THINK OF THE SHOULDERS GOING BACK AND DOWN, AS THE WEIGHT IS TAKEN THROUGH THE ARMS_ THIS WILL HELP YOU TO AVOID USING YOUR BICEPS AND PECTORALS UNNECESSARILY.

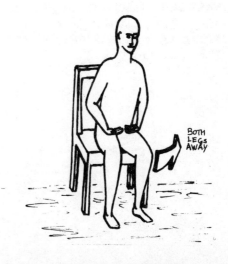

BOTH LEGS AWAY

• DESK WORK - KEYBOARDS AND WRITING ETC..

WHILE SEATED IN FRONT OF A TABLE OR DESK - POINT YOUR FINGERS TOWARDS THE FLOOR...
THEN - TURN YOUR HANDS INTO THE ANATOMICAL POSITION BY ROTATING YOUR THUMBS AROUND THE AXIS OF THE LITTLE FINGER (YOU MAY NOTICE THE ELBOWS COME INTO THE SIDES AS A RESULT)...
THEN - BRING BOTH HANDS UP TO REST (PALMS UP) ON THE WORK-SURFACE IN FRONT OF YOU...

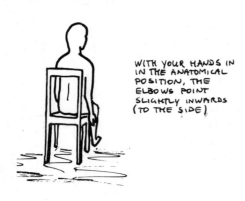

WITH YOUR HANDS IN IN THE ANATOMICAL POSITION, THE ELBOWS POINT SLIGHTLY INWARDS (TO THE SIDE)

NOW - USING THE IDEA OF THE THUMB AROUND THE LITTLE FINGER - TURN EACH HAND FROM SUPINE TO PRONE, AND BACK AGAIN (THAT IS - FROM PALMS UP TO PALMS DOWN, ETC)...

CAREFUL NOT TO LOSE THE FREEDOM IN THE ELBOWS BY FORCING IT IN EITHER DIRECTION...

THERE IS USUALLY AN EXTREME IN EITHER ONE DIRECTION OR THE OTHER SO - GO TO THE ONE MOST EASILY AVAILABLE, AND SEE HOW FAR YOU CAN GO WITHOUT FORCING IT...
THEN - GO TO THE OTHER SIDE ...
IN ORDER TO SUPINATE THE HAND FOR EXAMPLE - THE MUSCLES USED TO PRONATE MUST BE INHIBITED (THE NERVOUS SYSTEM ORGANIZES THE INTERACTION).

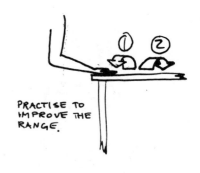

PRACTISE TO IMPROVE THE RANGE.

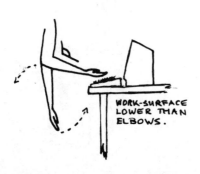

WORK-SURFACE LOWER THAN ELBOWS.

IF YOU FIND THAT THE WORK-SURFACE IS TOO HIGH (THE ELBOWS NEED TO BE AT THE SAME LEVEL, OR ABOVE, THE WORK-SURFACE) - THEN TRY RAISING THE CHAIR...
ALSO - AVOID LEANING IF AT ALL POSSIBLE - THIS NECESSITATES MORE MUSCULAR EFFORT.

· USING YOUR EYES WHILE TURNING .

WHILE SEATED — SLOWLY LOOK TOWARDS YOUR RIGHT SHOULDER
(AS ILLUSTRATED)···
THEN — ALLOW YOUR HEAD TO FOLLOW (SMOOTHLY)

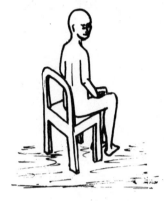

AVOID PUSHING — STOP AND THINK ABOUT IT —
THEN DIRECT AND CONTINUE···
IT IS NOT MUSCULAR EFFORT, BUT RELEASE
WHICH ACHIEVES THE RESULT···

THIS TIME — LOOK AHEAD OF YOU
WHILE TURNING YOUR TORSO···
AVOID STARING, AVOID PUSHING
WITH THE SHOULDERS, AND
AVOID TURNING YOUR HEAD···

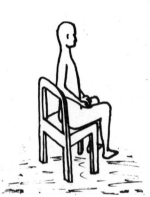

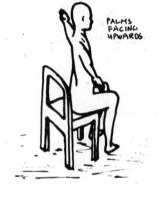

PALMS
FACING
UPWARDS

NOW — BRING BOTH ARMS OUT TO THE SIDE
(PALMS UP, ABOVE SHOULDER LEVEL)···
CONTINUING TO LOOK AHEAD — AND, ONCE
AGAIN, TURN YOUR TORSO TO THE RIGHT···
THEN — AS WITH ALL THE ACTIVITIES —
REPEAT ON THE OTHER SIDE···

NOTICE THE TENDENCY TO USE THE LEGS.

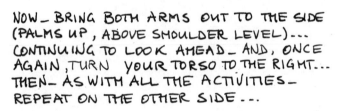

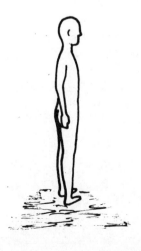

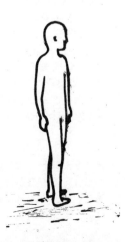

NOW IN STANDING — LOOK
AHEAD OF YOU, WHILE AT
THE SAME TIME, TURNING
THE UPPER PART OF THE
BODY (FROM THE HIPS)···
AVOID STARING AS THIS
STIFFENS THE NECK···

FINALLY — LOOKING AHEAD
OF YOU — TURN FROM THE
ANKLES (AGAIN WITHOUT
TURNING YOUR HEAD).

• MARKING TIME.

STANDING WITH YOUR FEET CLOSE TOGETHER (BUT NOT TOUCHING), AND, HAVING ACHIEVED BALANCE TO THE BEST OF YOUR SATISFACTION - ALLOW YOUR RIGHT KNEE TO MOVE (BEND.) FORWARD - THUS BENDING YOUR FOOT AT THE TOES AND RAISING YOUR HEEL OFF THE GROUND...
THEN - THINKING OF SENDING THE SAME HEEL TOWARDS THE FLOOR - ALLOW YOUR LEG TO STRAIGHTEN...

NOW - REPEAT THE INSTRUCTIONS ON THE OTHER SIDE.

NEXT - WHILE MAINTAINING THE DIRECTION TO GO UP - PROCEED TO THE POINT WHERE YOUR RIGHT HEEL IS RETURNING TO THE GROUND...
THEN - AT THE SAME TIME - LENGTHEN YOUR LEFT THIGH TO BEND THAT KNEE, AND RAISING THE LEFT HEEL OFF THE GROUND (AND BENDING YOUR FOOT AT THE TOES)...
CONTINUE THE ACTIVITY UNTIL A STEADY PACE IS ESTABLISHED, WITHOUT LIFTING YOUR FEET COMPLETELY OFF THE FLOOR.

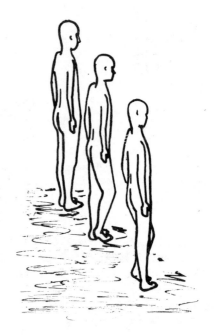

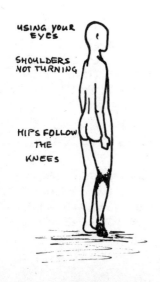

USING YOUR EYES

SHOULDERS NOT TURNING

HIPS FOLLOW THE KNEES

THIS TIME - CARRY OUT THE SAME INSTRUCTIONS - BUT ALLOW THE RIGHT HIP TO FOLLOW YOUR RIGHT KNEE, AND THEN THE LEFT HIP TO FOLLOW YOUR LEFT KNEE (IN A TWISTING ACTION)...
IN ADDITION TO THIS - LOOK AHEAD OF YOU - WHILE AVOIDING MOVEMENT OF THE SHOULDERS

FINALLY - COME A LITTLE MORE ON TO YOUR HEELS - AND TAKE A FEW STEPS BACKWARDS - THEN, WITHOUT PAUSING, WALK FORWARD.

• WALKING.

STANDING AS BEFORE – ALLOW YOUR HEAD TO ACT AS A BALANCER,
WHILE THE HEELS SUPPORT YOUR WEIGHT...
THEN – THINK OF ONE OF YOUR HEELS (THE LEFT HEEL FOR
EXAMPLE)...
AND – WHILE ALLOWING YOUR THOUGHT TO SHIFT THE WEIGHT
OVER TOWARDS THE LEFT HEEL – LENGTHEN AND WIDEN AT THE
SAME TIME...
THEN – AS YOUR RIGHT KNEE FREES FORWARD, AND YOUR RIGHT
HIP FOLLOWS – ALLOW THE CONTRAROTATION OF ARMS AND
HIPS TO TAKE PLACE, BRINGING THE RIGHT FOOT OFF THE
GROUND, INITIATING FORWARD LOCOMOTION...
NOW CONTINUE WALKING IN THIS MANNER – WHILE LOOKING
AHEAD OF YOU – PREVENT THE HEAD FROM TURNING TOWARDS
THE RIGHT OR LEFT...

OBSERVE HOW THE CONTRAROTATION ENERGISES THE WALK,
AND HOW ESSENTIAL IS THE FREEDOM OF THE SPINAL COLUMN,
FOR IT TO TAKE PLACE EFFORTLESSLY...

THE NEXT STAGE – WOULD BE TO WALK AS YOU NORMALLY
DO, AND THEN TAKE NOTE OF HOW THIS ACTION EXISTS AS
PART OF THE MOVEMENT.

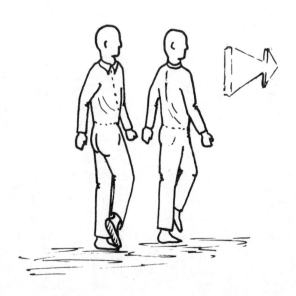

· BACK SUPPORT AND WHISPERED AH.

INVITE YOUR SEATED PUPIL TO MOVE DEEPER INTO THE CHAIR, BY USING BOTH HANDS ON THE SIDES OF THE SEAT — AND/OR — WALKING (ROCKING FROM SIDE TO SIDE) ON THE SITTING BONES...
THEN — PLACE A SUPPORT (TELEPHONE BOOK, CIGAR BOX ETC) AT SHOULDER-BLADE LEVEL, BEING CAREFUL NOT TO PUSH FORWARD...
NOW — RATHER THAN SAYING THINGS LIKE .. "COME BACK INTO YOUR BACK" — ALLOW THE PUPIL TO MOVE (PIVOT) AS ONE PIECE FROM THE HIPS .. "LIKE THE LID OF A BOX ON ITS HINGE...

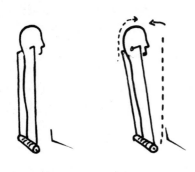

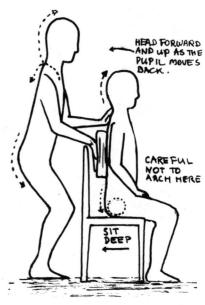

HEAD FORWARD AND UP AS THE PUPIL MOVES BACK.

CAREFUL NOT TO ARCH HERE

SIT DEEP

THE SITTING BONES TAKING THE WEIGHT — SHOULDERS BACK AND DOWN — HEAD FORWARD AND UP, ETC,. STERNUM NOT PULLED DOWN. ALL CONTRIBUTE TO COMING UP IN FRONT

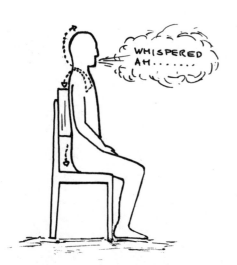

WHISPERED AH.......

NOW — ASK YOUR PUPIL TO DO A WHISPERED AH, AND USE IT TO OBSERVE UNNECESSARY DOWNWARD PULLING AS HE OR SHE IS BREATHING OUT.

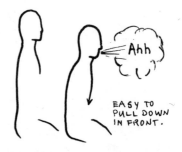

Ahh

EASY TO PULL DOWN IN FRONT.

· THE ATLANTO-OCCIPITAL JOINT, AND DISCOVERING IT'S RANGE.

WHILE SEATED, AND POINTING YOUR FINGERS TOWARDS THE FLOOR—
BEND AT THE ELBOW TO RAISE EACH HAND (IN TURN) TO
BETWEEN THE MASTOID PROCESSES (UNDER EACH EAR), AND THE
MANDIBLE OR JAW BONE...

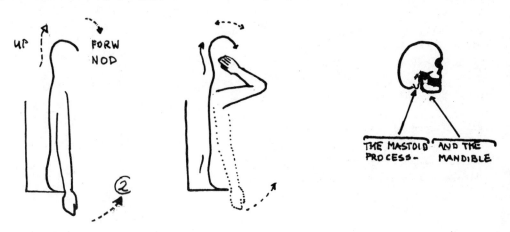

THE MASTOID PROCESS— AND THE MANDIBLE

NOW— GENTLY NOD YOUR HEAD, WHILE AT THE SAME TIME, OBSERVING
THE QUALITY OF THE MOVEMENT...

THIS TIME— BRING YOUR INDEX FINGER
UP TO UNDER THE NOSE AND
RESTING ON YOUR TOP LIP...
THEN— MOVE THE FINGER TO NOD YOUR
HEAD FORWARD— WHILE AT THE
SAME TIME TO STIMULATE A BACK
AND UPWARD MOVEMENT, OFF THE
ATLANTO-OCCIPITAL JOINT

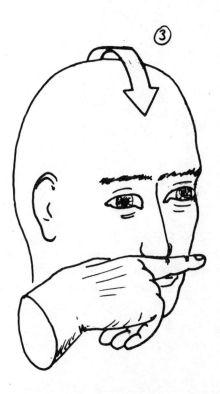

FORWARD AND UP
INVOLVING BACK
AND UP AND OFF
THE ATLANTO-
OCCIPITAL JOINT
DECOMPRESSING
THE SPINE

· WIDENING, BY PULLING TO THE ELBOWS.

WHILE SEATED — SLOWLY BRING BOTH
HANDS UP TO REST ON THE UPPER
PART OF YOUR CHEST, WITH
FINGERS ON YOUR COLLAR-BONES ...

NOW_ WHILE THINKING OF YOUR
SHOULDERS GOING BACK AND DOWN_
PULL TO THE ELBOWS (OR_ SEND
YOUR ELBOWS BACK AND AWAY
FROM YOUR WRISTS/HANDS)...

THEN_ALLOW YOUR HANDS TO
FOLLOW AFTER THE ELBOWS,
MOVING ACROSS THE CHEST AS
YOUR SHOULDERS WIDEN.

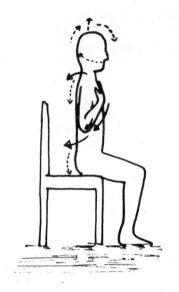

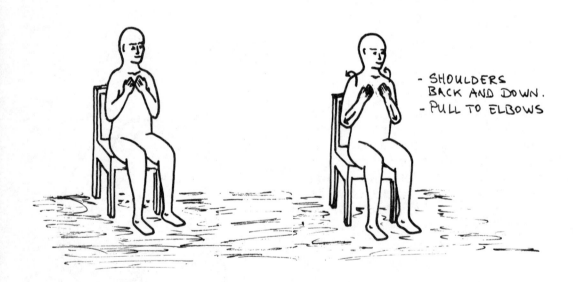

- SHOULDERS
BACK AND DOWN.
- PULL TO ELBOWS

CAREFUL AS YOU BRING BOTH HANDS UP AND ON TO YOUR
CHEST — IT IS VERY EASY TO RAISE THE SHOULDERS.
EXPERIENCE THE WEIGHT OF THE SHOULDERS GOING AWAY
FROM YOUR EARS (HEAD FORWARD AND UP).

• HANDS ON THE BACK OF A CHAIR.

WHILE SEATED — BRING BOTH HANDS UP TO REST (PALMS UP) ON THE BACK OF A CHAIR PLACED IN FRONT OF YOU...

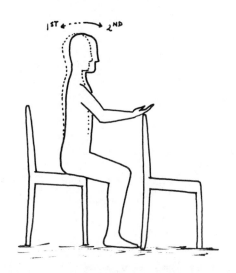

THEN— ALLOWING YOUR HEAD TO ACT AS A BALANCER, AND YOUR WEIGHT TO BE TAKEN BY THE SITTING-BONES — THINK OF YOUR ELBOWS GOING BACK AND DOWN...
NEXT—BEGIN ROCKING BACK AND FORTH (HINGING FROM YOUR SITTING-BONES), AND FREEING THE UPPER PART OF THE CHEST AND SHOULDERS...
NOW— THINK OF THE CONNECTION BETWEEN YOUR FINGERS AND THE BASE OF THE SPINE...

THEN— TURN BOTH HANDS (THUMBS AROUND LITTLE FINGERS, AND PALMS TOWARDS THE FLOOR)...
NOW— TAKE THE BACK OF THE CHAIR BETWEEN YOUR THUMBS AND STRAIGHT FINGERS.
FINALLY— DIRECT YOUR THUMBS TOWARDS THE GROUND IN ORDER TO STRAIGHTEN THE WRISTS...

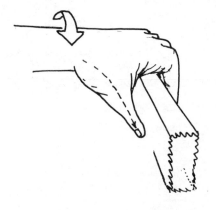

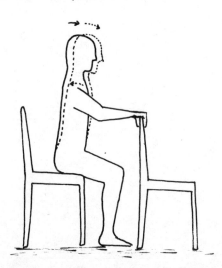

ONCE AGAIN— ROCK GENTLY BACK IN ORDER TO FREE YOUR HIPS ...
AND THEN— AS THOUGH YOUR TORSO WERE ADVANCING BETWEEN YOUR SHOULDERS (FREEING THE RIBS)— ROCK GENTLY FORWARD...

NEXT TIME—REPEAT THE ABOVE INSTRUCTIONS WHILE STANDING IN MONKEY...
LOOK FOR FREEDOM BETWEEN YOUR FINGERS AND BASE OF THE SPINE/HEELS, THROUGHOUT.

TERM THREE
SECOND HALF

• SHOULDERS WIDENING.

WHEN THE NECK MUSCLES ARE ALLOWED TO BE FREE FROM
PULLING THE HEAD BACK AND DOWN,
THE HEAD CAN THEN BALANCE (NODDING FORWARD AND UP)
MORE EFFECTIVELY.
THEN CONDITIONS ARE MORE SUITABLE FOR THE BACK TO
LENGTHEN ...
WHILE AT THE SAME TIME _ WIDENING THE UPPER PART OF
THE BACK AND CHEST BY SENDING THE SHOULDERS BACK
AND DOWN ...

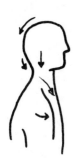 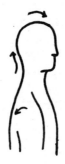 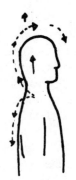

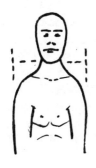

F.M. WAS KNOWN TO
HAVE SAID TO HIS
PUPILS _ " BACK AND
DOWN WITH THE
SHOULDERS, TO WIDEN
THE UPPER PART OF THE
BACK".

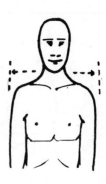

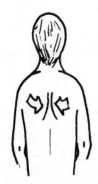

A COMMON MISTAKE _ IS TO TIGHTEN
BETWEEN THE SHOULDER _ BLADES, IN
THE BELIEF THAT THIS WOULD HELP TO
"STRAIGHTEN THE SHOULDERS" _
INSTEAD, THIS WILL ONLY SERVE TO
NARROW THE UPPER BACK AND CHEST
EVEN FURTHER.

• SHOULDERS WIDENING (CONTINUED).

STANDING, WITH YOUR WEIGHT
OVER THE HEELS, AND YOUR
HEAD ACTING AS A BALANCER—
POINT YOUR FINGERS TOWARDS
THE FLOOR...
THEN— TURN YOUR HANDS INTO
THE ANATOMICAL POSITION (BY
MOVING THE THUMB AROUND THE
AXIS OF THE LITTLE FINGER)...
NOW— WITH THE ELBOWS TENDING
TO POINT INWARDS (TOWARDS THE
RIBS) — ALLOW THE MOVEMENT OF
THE RIBS TO HELP WITH YOUR
DIRECTIONS FOR THE SHOULDERS
TO GO BACK AND DOWN, WHILE
WIDENING AT THE SAME TIME.

THE ACTION OF THE LOWER RIBS
IS LIKE THE SIDEWAYS MOVEMENT
OF A BUCKET HANDLE.

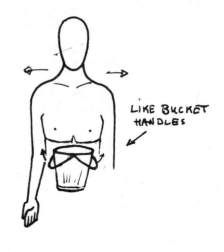

LIKE BUCKET
HANDLES

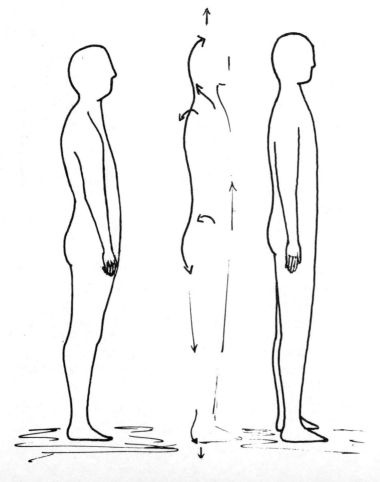

USING YOUR HEELS
TO TAKE YOUR
WEIGHT— RELEASE
THE NECK MUSCLES
TO FREE THE HEAD
FORWARD AND UP...
THEN ALLOW YOUR
PELVIS TO GO
BACK AND DOWN
(DROPPING YOUR
BOTTOM), AND
YOUR SHOULDERS
ALSO TO GO BACK
AND DOWN
(DROPPING YOUR
SHOULDER BLADES)...
NOW LENGTHENING
IN BOTH DIRECTIONS
CAN TAKE PLACE.

LENGTHENING AND
WIDENING.

• HANDS ON THE TABLE (LIKE FEET ON THE GROUND).

STANDING IN MONKEY IN FRONT OF THE TEACHING TABLE — TURN BOTH HANDS INTO THE ANATOMICAL POSITION (WIDENING)... THEN — TAKING CARE 'OT TO PULL THE SHOULDERS IN OR LIFT THEM USING YOUR ELTOIDS — BRING BOTH HANDS UP TO REST (FINGERS CLOSED AND PALMS DOWN) ON THE TABLE...

NOW — SEND YOUR KNEES FORWARD, WHILE AT THE SAME TIME TAKING SOME OF THE WEIGHT ON TO YOUR HANDS... THEN — USE (THE HEELS OF) YOUR HANDS, IN THE SAME WAY AS YOU USE THE HEELS (OF YOUR FEET) TO DIRECT FROM. YOU ARE NOW USING THE HEELS OF BOTH HANDS — AND FEET AS THOUGH YOU WERE FOUR-FOOTED, HIPS AND SHOULDERS ACTING SIMILARLY...

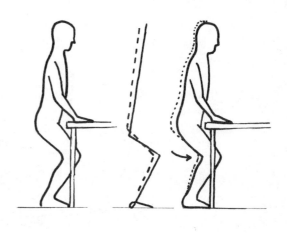

NEXT TIME — WHEN YOU BRING BOTH HANDS TO REST ON THE TABLE — SPREAD YOUR FINGERS APART... THEN — SENDING YOUR KNEES FORWARD — BRING SOME OF YOUR WEIGHT ON TO THE HANDS...

NOTICE THE WAY IN WHICH YOUR WEIGHT IS DISTRIBUTED, AND COMPARE THE QUALITY OF YOUR MOVEMENT WITH THE PREVIOUS WAY...

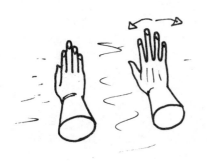

FINALLY — AS BEFORE (WITH THE FINGERS TOGETHER) — USE THE HEELS OF YOUR HANDS TO DIRECT FROM... THEN — POINTING YOUR FINGERS AWAY — EXTEND YOUR WRISTS.

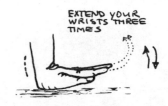

EXTEND YOUR WRISTS THREE TIMES

• HANDS ON THE TABLE (CONTINUED).

AGAIN — STANDING IN MONKEY IN FRONT OF THE TEACHING TABLE, WITH BOTH HANDS (PALMS DOWN) RESTING ON IT — ARCH YOUR HANDS...
THEN — AS BEFORE — SEND YOUR KNEES FORWARD TO BRING YOUR WEIGHT ONTO BOTH HANDS...

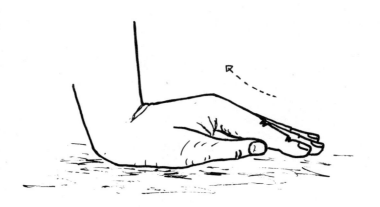

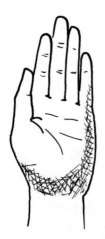

NOTICE HOW THE WEIGHT IS DISTRIBUTED FROM THE HEELS OF THE HANDS AROUND TO THE OUTSIDES...
AT THE SAME TIME — THE WEIGHT ON EACH FOOT IS DISTRIBUTED THE SAME WAY, FROM BOTH HEELS — OUT TOWARDS THE OUTSIDES...

THIS ENABLES WIDENING ACROSS THE UPPER PART OF THE BACK, CHEST, AND SHOULDERS TO TAKE PLACE MORE EASILY.

• SHOULDERS AND ARMS.

WHILE STANDING — POINT YOUR
FINGERS TOWARDS THE FLOOR,
AND OPEN BOTH HANDS...
THEN — TURN YOUR HANDS INTO
THE ANATOMICAL POSITION
(THUMBS AROUND LITTLE
FINGERS)...
NOW — ALLOW THE WEIGHT OF
THE ARMS TO LENGTHEN THE
DELTOID MUSCLES...
NEXT — BEND AT THE ELBOWS
WHILE AT THE SAME TIME —
THINKING OF THE ELBOWS
GOING TOWARDS THE FLOOR...
NOW THAT YOUR HANDS ARE
AT SHOULDER HEIGHT —
SEND THEM AWAY FROM
EACHOTHER (WIDENING THE
SPACE BETWEEN THEM)...
FINALLY — ALLOW GRAVITY TO
BRING YOUR HANDS BACK
DOWN BY YOUR SIDES, WHILE
ATTENDING TO THE WIDTH
BETWEEN THE SHOULDERS.

TIGHTENING IN THE DELTOIDS
LIMITS THE FREE HANGING
OF THE ARMS FROM THE
SHOULDERS.

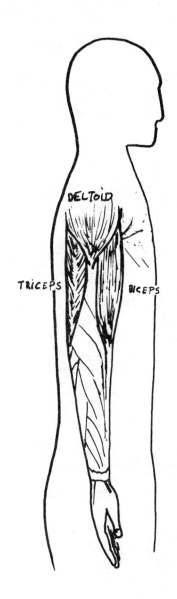

DELTOID

TRICEPS

BICEPS

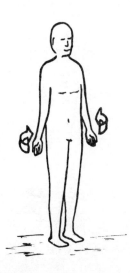
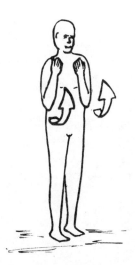
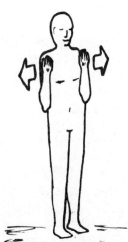

• SHOULDERS AND ARMS (CONTINUED).

ONCE AGAIN — WHILE STANDING — POINT YOUR FINGERS (ONE HAND AT A TIME) TOWARDS THE FLOOR, ALLOWING GRAVITY TO HELP YOUR DIRECTIONS TO LENGTHEN THE ARM...

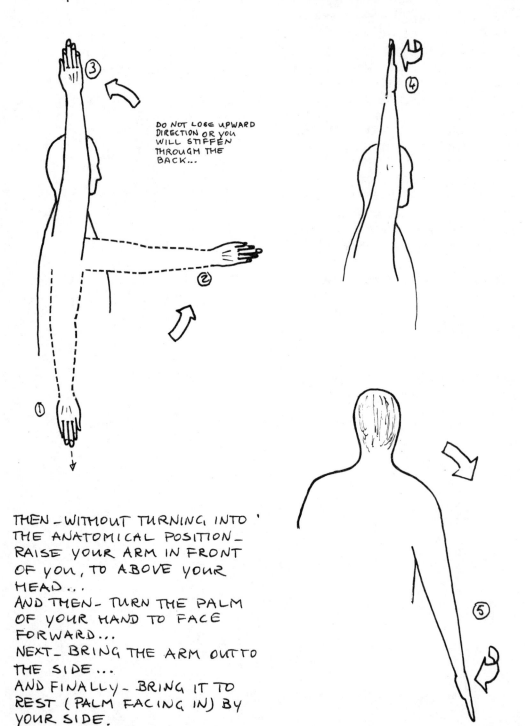

DO NOT LOSE UPWARD DIRECTION OR YOU WILL STIFFEN THROUGH THE BACK...

THEN — WITHOUT TURNING INTO THE ANATOMICAL POSITION — RAISE YOUR ARM IN FRONT OF YOU, TO ABOVE YOUR HEAD...
AND THEN — TURN THE PALM OF YOUR HAND TO FACE FORWARD...
NEXT — BRING THE ARM OUT TO THE SIDE...
AND FINALLY — BRING IT TO REST (PALM FACING IN) BY YOUR SIDE.

· HANDS ON SHOULDERS.

STANDING IN MONKEY AT
THE BACK OF YOUR
SEATED PUPIL — BRING
BOTH HANDS UP TO REST
ON HIS/HER SHOULDERS,
AS WITH HANDS ON THE
TABLE...
THEN — SENDING YOUR
KNEES SLIGHTLY FORWARD —
MAKE CONTACT WITH THE
HEELS OF YOUR HANDS
(AND FEET)...
NOW — EVEN THOUGH YOU
COULD NOT LIFT YOUR
PUPIL STRAIGHT UP —
DIRECT AS IF YOU COULD...
FINALLY — COME BACK INTO
VERTICAL...

THROUGHOUT THIS WORK —
ATTEND TO — HEAD FORWARD
AND UP — HIPS BACK AND
DOWN — SHOULDERS BACK
AND DOWN — KNEES FORWARD
AND ELBOWS BACK ...

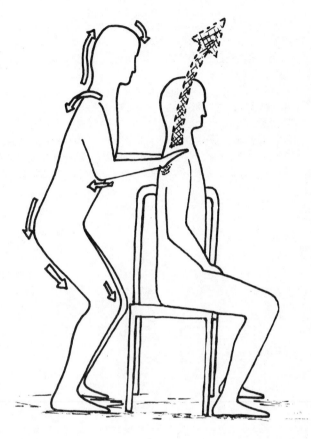

PUPIL THINKS OF
COMING BACK

TEACHER STANDS
PUPIL UP

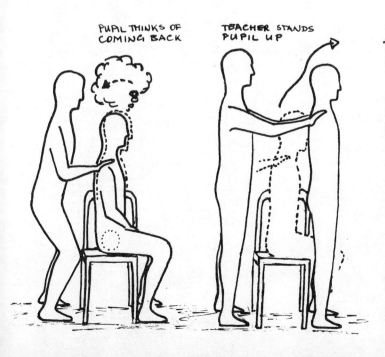

THIS TIME — AFTER YOU
HAVE CONTACTED THE
PUPILS SHOULDERS —
ALLOW HIM/HER TO
USE YOUR HANDS TO
HELP REDUCE ANY
UNNECESSARY TENSION
IN THE LEGS ...
NOW CONNECT THIS EXTRA
WEIGHT WITH THE GROUND
UNDER YOUR HEELS ...
FINALLY — IN ONE EVEN
MOVEMENT — TAKE THE
PUPIL BACK, VERY
SLIGHTLY BEYOND
VERTICAL, AND MOVE
(PUSH, SHOVE) INTO
STANDING.

• MONKEY AND CHAIR WORK WITH A PUPIL.

BEGIN BY STANDING BEHIND YOUR (STANDING) PUPIL...
THEN – GO INTO MONKEY, AND BRING BOTH HANDS UP TO UNDER
THE PUPIL'S ARMS – THE HEELS OF YOUR HANDS TOWARDS THE
BACK...
NOW – ALLOW THE PUPIL TO USE YOUR SUPPORT TO FREE THE
ANKLES FROM UNNECESSARY TENSING – (COMING BACK SLIGHTLY)...
THEN – AVOID ANY PUSHING – AND – YOU GO INTO A DEEPER MONKEY,
AS YOUR PUPIL GOES INTO MONKEY (USING HIS/HER HEELS TO
TAKE THEIR WEIGHT – AND DIRECT UP FROM)...
FINALLY – COME BACK INTO VERTICAL (USING KNEES FORWARD)...

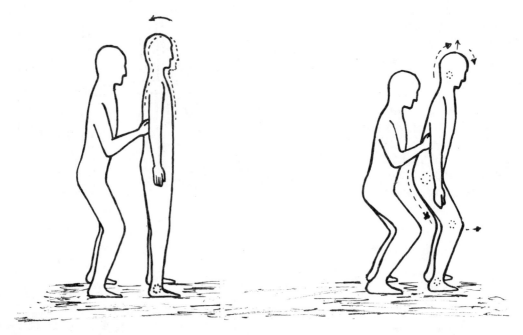

THE NEXT STAGE SHOULD BE
RESERVED FOR PUPILS WITH
SOME EXPERIENCE OF THE
ALEXANDER TECHNIQUE.

WITH A CHAIR (OR STOOL)
PLACED BETWEEN YOU AND
THE PUPIL – FOLLOW THE
PREVIOUS INSTRUCTIONS, AND
GUIDE THE PUPIL INTO THE
CHAIR –

REMEMBER THAT A GOOD "UP"
DEPENDS ON A GOOD "GROUND".

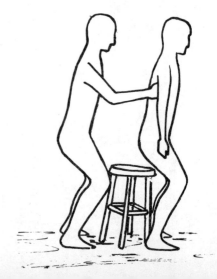

- BODY TWISTING UNDER A STATIONARY HEAD.

FIRST – WHILE SITTING IN A CHAIR – LOOK AHEAD OF YOU, FOCUSING ON AN OBJECT... THEN – WITHOUT PUSHING WITH YOUR LEGS – TURN TO THE RIGHT, WHILE THE HEAD REMAINS STATIONARY... AND THEN – TO THE LEFT...

TAKE CARE NOT TO PULL YOUR OPPOSITE SHOULDER AROUND IN AN ATTEMPT AT ACHIEVING A "SUCCESSFUL" TURN ...

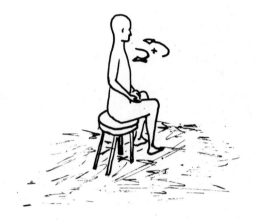

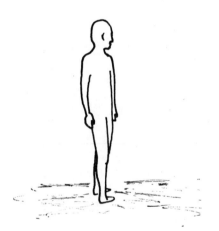

THIS TIME – WHILE STANDING – REPEAT THE ABOVE INSTRUCTIONS, TURNING FROM THE ANKLES – WHILE LOOKING (NOT STARING) AHEAD OF YOU, AND KEEPING THE HEAD STATIONARY...

THIS COMPLEX MOVEMENT OF ROTATION AROUND THE SPINE – USES THE MUSCLES ON ALTERNATE SIDES AS YOU TURN TO THE RIGHT, AND THEN TO THE LEFT ...

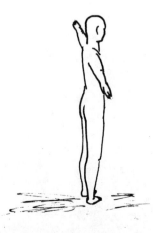

ONCE AGAIN – WHILE STANDING – POINT YOUR FINGERS TOWARDS THE FLOOR ... THEN – BRING YOUR ARMS UP AND OUT TO THE SIDES (PALMS FACING UPWARDS)... NOW – TURN TO THE RIGHT (USING THE ARMS AS AN EXTENSION OF THE SPINE) AND THEN TO THE LEFT.

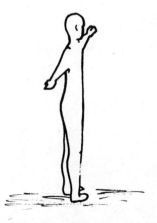

· TURNING THE HIPS.

STANDING WITH YOUR FEET CLOSE TOGETHER, BUT NOT
TOUCHING. LOOK AHEAD OF YOU (NOT STARING)...
THEN _ FREEING YOUR RIGHT KNEE FORWARD _ TURN YOUR
PELVIS TOWARDS THE LEFT, WHILE KEEPING THE UPPER
PART OF YOUR BODY FREE FROM FOLLOWING THE TURN...
AND THEN _ REPEAT THE INSTRUCTIONS ON THE OTHER
SIDE...
NEXT _ CONTINUE THE MOVEMENTS INTO A SMOOTH TURNING
FROM SIDE TO SIDE (NOT AGGRESSIVELY TWISTING)...

FINALLY _ MOVE YOUR HIPS FROM SIDE TO SIDE WITHOUT
BENDING AT THE KNEES, BUT NOT TIGHTENING IN THE LEGS
TO DO SO.

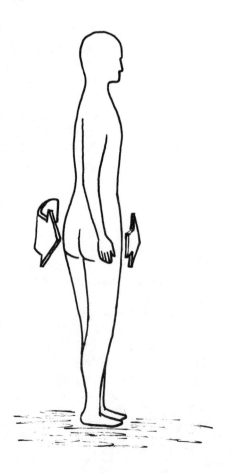

• HIPS AND SHOULDERS.

BEGIN BY LOOKING AT AN OBJECT IN FRONT OF YOU...
THEN - TURN YOUR HIPS TO THE RIGHT...
AND NOW - TURN YOUR SHOULDERS TO THE LEFT...BY POINTING
THE FINGERS OF YOUR RIGHT HAND TOWARDS YOUR LEFT
FOOT...
TAKE CARE NOT TO PUSH WITH THE SHOULDER - OR TO TURN
YOUR HEAD IN SYMPATHY -

NOW - FOLLOW THE INSTRUCTIONS ON THE OTHER SIDE...

NEXT - BEGIN WITH A FLOWING MOVEMENT OF THE HIPS...
THEN - INTRODUCE THE SHOULDERS (BY POINTING THE FINGERS),
AND CONTINUE IN A FLOWING CONTRAROTATION OF THE HIPS
AND SHOULDERS...

THIS TIME - BEGIN THE ACTION WITH THE SHOULDERS
(FOLLOWING THE FINGERS)...

FINALLY - TAKE THE MOVEMENT INTO WALKING (POINTING AT
THE FORWARD TOE).

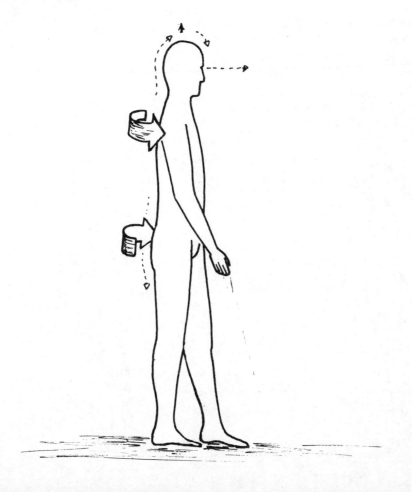

• GOING UP.. ON YOUR TOES.

WHILE IN MONKEY BEHIND YOUR
PUPIL _ BRING BOTH HANDS UP
ON TO THE PUPIL'S SIDES
(JUST ABOVE ELBOW LEVEL) _
WITH THE HEELS OF YOUR HANDS
CONTACTING THE BACK...
NOW _ WITH THE PUPIL'S FEET
CLOSE TOGETHER, BUT NOT
TOUCHING _ ENCOURAGE HIM/HER
TO SEND THE WEIGHT _ FROM THE
HEELS _ AROUND THE OUTSIDES
OF THE FEET ...
WHILE AT THE SAME TIME _ TO
ALLOW THE FORWARD AND UP
OF THE HEAD _ TO CARRY
HIM/HER ON TO THE TOES (AS
THOUGH MOVING IN ONE PIECE...

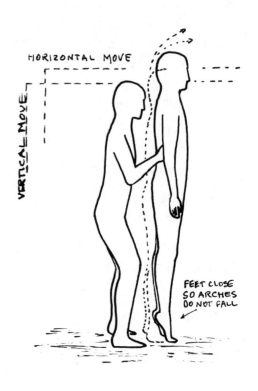

HORIZONTAL MOVE

VERTICAL MOVE

FEET CLOSE
SO ARCHES
DO NOT FALL

ALTERNATIVELY _ ALLOW YOUR
PUPIL TO COME BACK INTO YOUR
HANDS. AND WHILE YOU CONTINUE
RESISTING ANY BACKWARDS
MOVEMENT _ THE PUPIL IS
OBLIGED TO DIRECT, AND GO
UP ON HIS/HER TOES .

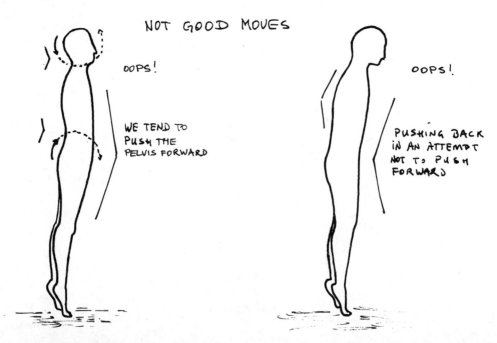

NOT GOOD MOVES

OOPS!

WE TEND TO
PUSH THE
PELVIS FORWARD

OOPS!

PUSHING BACK
IN AN ATTEMPT
NOT TO PUSH
FORWARD

• UP ON YOUR TOES IN MONKEY.

STANDING WITH YOUR FEET WIDER APART THAN REQUIRED FOR THE PREVIOUS ACTIVITY...
THEN — BALANCING OVER YOUR HEELS (AND OUTSIDES OF FEET) — HEAD FORWARD, KNEES FORWARD, HIPS BACK — GO INTO MONKEY...

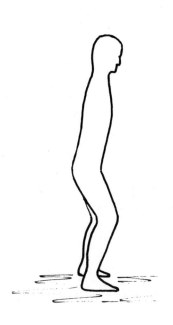

NOW — DIRECTING YOUR HEAD MORE FORWARD AND UP — ALLOW YOUR WEIGHT TO MOVE AROUND THE OUTSIDES OF THE FEET, FROM YOUR HEELS TO YOUR TOES...
AND — AS IN THE PREVIOUS GAME — MOVE VERTICALLY FORWARD AND HORIZONTALLY UP...

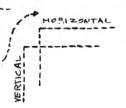

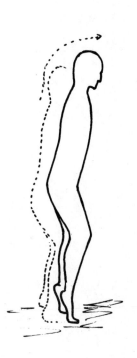

BE CAREFUL NOT TO ALLOW THIS TO HAPPEN...

SIMPLY PUSHING THE KNEES FORWARD — WITHOUT THE FORWARD AND UP TO CARRY YOU UPWARDS AND OVER THE TOES.

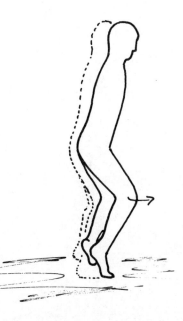

OOPS! NOT GOOD.

SPIRALS

145

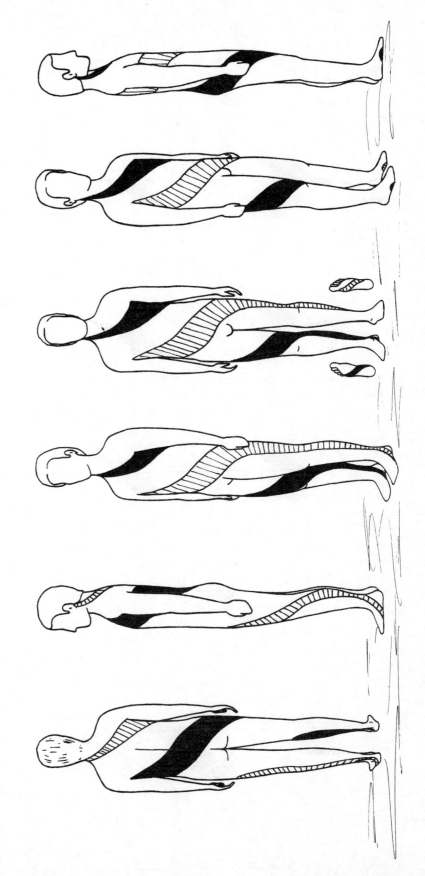

- S P I R A L S -

IT IS USEFUL TO THINK OF RELEASING SPIRALLY (BOTH YOU AND YOUR PUPIL).

THE FOLLOWING CAN BE SEEN AS A PRACTICAL WORKING MODEL, AND IF YOU

HOLD THE PAGE UP TO THE LIGHT YOU CAN SEE HOW THE RIGHT AND LEFT, OR

FRONT AND BACK SPIRALS FIT TOGETHER (DOUBLE SPIRAL).

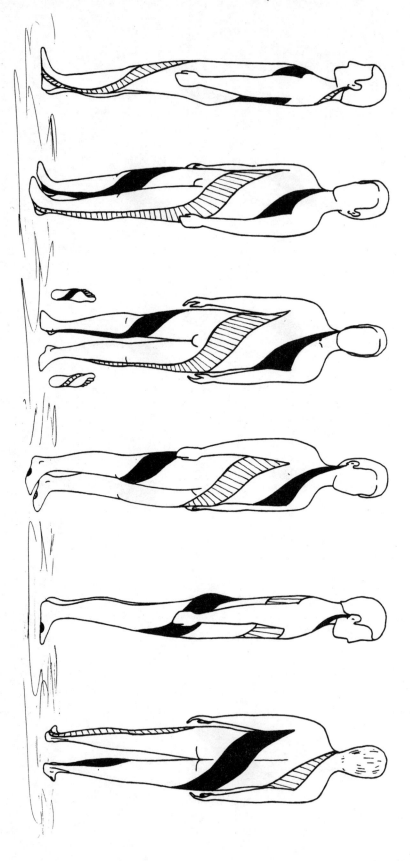

Index of directed activities